EXECUTIVE COMPENSATION

Guidelines for Healthcare

Leaders and Trustees

EXECUTIVE COMPENSATION

Guidelines for Healthcare Leaders and Trustees

edited by Thomas P. Flannery

Health Administration Press

ACHE Management Series

Your board, staff, or clients may also benefit from this book's insight. For more information on quantity discounts, contact the Health Administration Press Marketing Manager at (312) 424-9470.

This publication is intended to provide accurate and authoritative information in regard to the subject matter covered. It is sold, or otherwise provided, with the understanding that the publisher is not engaged in rendering professional services. If professional advice or other expert assistance is required, the services of a competent professional should be sought.

The statements and opinions contained in this book are strictly those of the author(s) and do not represent the official positions of the American College of Healthcare Executives or of the Foundation of the American College of Healthcare Executives.

06   05   04   03   02   5   4   3   2   1

Library of Congress Cataloging-in-Publication Data

Arthur Andersen LLP.
    Executive compensation : guidelines for healthcare leaders and trustees / by Andersen LLP ; edited by Thomas P. Flannery.
        p. cm.
    Includes bibliographical references and index.
    ISBN 1-56793-184-7 (alk.paper)
    1. Hospital administrators—Salaries, etc.   I. Flannery, Thomas P. (Thomas Patrick), 1949–   II. Title.

RA971.A826 2002
331.2'813621—dc21   2002017128

The paper used in this publication meets the minimum requirements of American National Standard for Information Sciences-Permanence of Paper for Printed Library Materials, ANSI Z39.48-1984.™

Acquisitions editor: Marcy McKay; Project manager: Cami Cacciatore; Cover design: Betsy Pérez

Health Administration Press
A division of the
Foundation of the American College of Healthcare Executives
1 North Franklin Street, Suite 1700
Chicago, IL 60606-3491
(312) 424-2800

Table of Contents

Acknowledgements

THE AMERICAN COLLEGE of Healthcare Executives approached me to prepare this book in early 2000. Since that time, I have worked with a number of individuals who have gone out of their way to ensure that I received the support necessary to complete this book.

Foremost, I would like to thank the many executives and board member clients that I have worked with over the years. This group experiences, day-to-day, the challenges of providing an environment for physicians and other healthcare workers to deliver services to our families, to our friends, and to members of our communities. Each board member and executive stands on the front line, balancing all public healthcare policy, cost, service, and quality challenges that affect us all.

Several colleagues and friends have also provided significant help and insight. Kathy Vestal, Deborah Proctor, Howard Chase, Allan Cohen, Al Cappelloni, John Dirlam, John Gunn, Gene LeBlonde, Lee Pearlman, and Clark Taylor have each provided insights that have helped to shape this book.

I especially want to thank Bruce Benesh for providing the encouragement to complete this guidebook. Kent Graham went beyond the call of duty in reading each and every chapter and provided an important quality check for this book. Alexandra Lajoux provided invaluable editorial support with the manuscript, making the chapters flow. Amber Peters facilitated communications among the numerous parties involved in this project, providing valuable administrative skills.

Without Bruce Meyer, this book would not have been possible. Bruce was always able to set aside time to work with me to sharpen the outline, identify contributors, and critique.

Last but not least, I thank our distinguished contributors for making this book possible. It has been an honor to serve as their editor, and a privilege to work as their colleague.

Introduction

TODAY, COMPENSATION POSES a distinct challenge to the healthcare field—one that applies both to the executives' pay and the board members approving it. In the currently competitive environment, institutions want to attract and retain the best talent, which often means paying "top dollar." At the same time, however, institutions and executives want to show communities that they are putting community needs first, which often means showing compensation restraint.

Compensation restraint is also being encouraged by external trends.

- The so-called "managed care" movement, with its focus on consumer price savings, lowered the profitability of the major players in the field—which includes insurers, providers, and physicians—and forced consolidations and/or networks among them. Managed care in some sectors brought an inevitable and involuntary decline in quality, and a consequent drop in the morale of providers.

- Over the past five years, a series of tax bills have directly or indirectly affected executive compensation. The 1996 Taxpayer Bill of Rights, through subsequent regulation (notably in 1999), placed restrictions on senior executive pay in nonprofits. In 1997, the Balanced Budget Act reduced Medicare payments for most hospital services, putting financial pressures on hospitals that in some cases have led to pay conservatism. The 2001 Economic Growth and Tax Relief Reconciliation Act increased contribution limits for pension plans, inspiring some organizations to allocate more pay into pensions rather than into current compensation.

As a result of changes like these, healthcare leaders can find themselves in a bind—feeling both an upward pressure on pay aspirations and a downward pressure on pay levels. Different healthcare institutions respond in different ways to such pressures, based in part on the variety of market forces they face.

In a study of healthcare executive compensation based on the most recent 990 forms, Andersen found a wide range of total compensation for all positions it studied, including the positions of chief executive officer (CEO), chief operating officer (COO), chief financial officer (CFO), senior human resources officer, and the vice president of patient relations. In analyzing these differences, Andersen confirmed that a variety of factors can influence these differences in compensation levels—notably location (urban versus rural). Other factors include level of responsibility of the position and strategic business goals and objectives.

Given the importance of pay in meeting the needs of executives, institutions and communities, and given the wide range of pay practices possible, there is clearly a need for guidance in this area. To provide such guidance, Andersen has joined with the American College for Healthcare Executives, to offer *Executive Compensation: Guidelines for Healthcare Leaders and Trustees*.

CHANGES IN THE HEALTHCARE FIELD

The timing of this book is good, and the cause is worthy. The talent pool in healthcare has diminished in recent decades. Other more lucrative fields are luring would-be healthcare executives away early in their careers. The career opportunities in other sectors, especially with the prospects of higher total compensation and stock options have also started to reshape the healthcare industry.

All these developments, taken together, are forcing organizations to use their financial resources ever more judiciously as they recruit and reward talent. The need to gain greater value for pay has affected organizations differently. Many for-profit organizations are tightening their compensation budgets. Conversely, many not-for-profits are expanding them, to bring compensation levels into a perceived "norm" defined by their for-profit competitors.

Yet even as healthcare organizations adjust to changing realities, some issues have not changed. The healthcare field, as always, still needs to develop its future generation of leaders. As part of this need, the field must find ways of rewarding them economically and professionally, to entice talented professionals in both management and medicine to stay in the healthcare profession.

All of these factors merge to create an environment where directors are challenged to strike a balance between their need to pay, their ability to pay, and their willingness to pay. For their part, executives must set their own clear expectations for compensation and then perform to the standards mutually agreed between themselves and board members.

This book addresses the many complex issues that must be considered by executives and board members as they work to reach agreement on compensation packages. Each chapter in this guidebook comes from professionals knowledgeable in the fields of both healthcare and compensation. Here are some highlights:

Chapter 1 sets a baseline for this book by explaining the role of the board in for-profit versus not-for-profit institutions, including the role of the chairman of the board and the chairman and members of the board compensation committee. The chapter then explains how the board's role relates to the setting of senior executive pay.

Chapter 2 discusses the basic elements of compensation—namely cash (including base salary, bonuses, and incentives), benefits, equity, and perquisites—and explains how they work together to make a full compensation package. It also explains the nuances of pay *timing* (short-term, long-term, deferred).

Chapter 3 gives an overview of some of the philosophical issues involved in pay, as well as the link between pay and performance, including a discussion of how to set performance indicators in a healthcare institution.

Chapter 4 explains how to ensure that compensation is "reasonable," and how to avoid sanctions levied against unreasonable pay (stemming from the 1996 tax law mentioned above). Chapter 5 offers technical guidance on ways to defer payment of income to help executives accumulate wealth.

Chapter 6 reviews the basic components of employment contracts, which the author recommends putting in writing. This chapter includes a change of control agreement as an appendix. Written by a successful "headhunter" in the healthcare field, Chapter 7 focuses on recruitment and retention.

Physician pay is the subject of Chapter 8, which offers "new ways to ensure that physicians receive compensation commensurate with the value of their service." The book closes in Chapter 9 with a guide to establishing positive media relations, complete with "ten tips" and more than a dozen "dos and don'ts."

These chapters raise and answer many important questions. Above all, they make one point abundantly clear: Whether an institution is small or large, for-profit or not-for-profit, compensation will be an extremely important issue that must be managed with great care.

Thomas P. Flannery, PH.D.

Setting Senior Executive Compensation Policies for Healthcare Institutions: Governance Foundations

Thomas P. Flannery

MOST LEADERS OF healthcare institutions have chosen their roles for nonfinancial reasons. The very business of healthcare—to provide health services to individuals and communities—calls upon humanity's deepest impulse: to help one's neighbor. Whether they are working for a large, for-profit, diversified healthcare empire, or a small, not-for-profit organization, senior executives deserve reward and recognition commensurate with their services. It is up to the board of directors (or trustees) to set a policy for determining the financial aspects of that reward.

This book provides information that both board members and senior officers can use to set executive compensation policies, focusing on several aspects of compensation:

- The elements of compensation, defining "reasonable compensation"
- Performance and pay
- Income deferral and wealth accumulation
- Employment contracts
- Recruitment of healthcare executives
- Physician compensation
- Establishing positive public relations

1

This opening chapter sets an overall context for these important concerns. It explains the basic role of the board of a healthcare institution, including the role of the chairman of the board and the chairman and members of the compensation committee. It then explains how this role relates to the setting of senior executive pay.

THE ROLE OF THE BOARD IN FOR-PROFIT VERSUS NOT-FOR-PROFIT INSTITUTIONS

The role of the board of a healthcare institution is to steer the institution in the correct direction. In the case of both for-profit and not-for-profit institutions, this is typically a public benefit imbedded in a mission statement. Both the for-profit and not-for-profit institutions serve their stakeholders. In the case of the for-profit institution, the primary stakeholders are the shareholders, whereas in the not-for-profit institution, the primary stakeholders are the beneficiaries of the institution's mission.

Director Duties by State Statute

Directors of both for-profit and not-for-profit corporations have duties according to state statutes of incorporation. Most state statutes say that a "corporation shall be managed under the direction of a board of directors."

Board members ensure that a corporation is well managed. They do this by selecting the right chief executive officer (CEO), by ensuring good succession planning for CEO and other senior officer positions, and by monitoring CEO and senior executive performance. These indeed are considered the most crucial responsibilities of boards—in addition to their basic responsibilities set forth by state statutes and by corporate bylaws.

At a minimum, as stated in most state statutes of incorporation, director approval is usually required for amendments to corporation bylaws, and recommendations to shareholders to amend articles of incorporation, dissolve the corporation, or sell or otherwise relinquish control of substantially all the assets of the corporation. In corporations that issue shares, directors are also responsible for the issuance of shares and declaration of dividends.

Contrasts Between For-Profit and Not-for-Profit Director Duties

The for-profit corporation director must serve the interests of shareholders. The director also has duties with respect to other constituencies, as described in state and federal laws, but because of the nature of the corporation, in general, shareholder interests must come first.

Internal Revenue Service rules as well as most state not-for-profit corporation laws require that to receive tax-exempt status, the charter of a not-for-profit corporation must describe its reason for being and its basic activities. Whereas a for-profit corporation may engage in any legal activity, the not-for-profit corporation must do only what furthers the purposes for which it was formed.

Duties of Care and Loyalty—and Relevance to Executive Compensation

The director has duties of care and loyalty under state statutes of incorporation. According to these statutes, the director must oversee the affairs of the corporation with due care, avoiding conflicts of interest in any particular transaction. In light of these duties, it is clear that directors of corporations *must have a careful process for establishing executive pay levels,* and they *must not be involved in setting pay if they have a conflict of interest.* These two points are developed more fully below.

In both for-profit and not-for-profit healthcare organizations, directors must establish a careful, independent process for determining executive pay. The remainder of this chapter describes best practices for establishing such a process. The findings presented here are based on my own work with the boards of healthcare institutions, and are confirmed by the latest findings of various authoritative sources.

ESTABLISHING A CAREFUL, INDEPENDENT PROCESS FOR SETTING EXECUTIVE PAY

So how, precisely, can a healthcare institution set a careful, independent process for setting pay? In my experience, there are two important cornerstones. One is an effective chairman of the board; the other is a compensation committee independent of management.

Most healthcare institutions separate the chairman and CEO role. This allows the chairman to evaluate CEO performance. In 1993, the American College of Healthcare Executives (ACHE) published *The Partnership Study: A Study of the Roles and Working Relationships of the Hospital Board Chairman, CEO, and Medical Staff President; Survey Findings.* Conducted jointly by ACHE, the American Hospital Association, the American Medical Association, and Ernst & Young LLP, this national study surveyed 1,200 randomly selected hospital board chairmen, CEOs, and medical staff presidents (elected leaders). The research "documented that board chairmen function to ensure quality healthcare, *evaluate the CEO's performance,* and develop the hospital's strategic plan" (ACHE 1993).

The chairman of the board can play an important role in the formation of an independent compensation committee. If the chairman is the CEO, then he or she should not serve on the committee. Rather, most governance experts believe the compensation committee should be composed entirely of independent outside directors. Although no U.S. federal law, state law, or stock exchange listing requires an all-independent compensation committee, many healthcare institution stakeholders expect this. This expectation is reflected in federal tax law—the U.S. Internal Revenue Code, under Section 162(m), sets a limit of $1 million on the deductibility of executive compensation, unless such compensation is awarded under a performance-based plan approved by an all-independent compensation committee. Further restrictions are found in the intermediate sanctions regulations discussed in Chapter 4 of this book.

By definition, a CEO is an insider and not independent. Therefore, it is not recommended that the CEO serve on the compensation committee (especially not to approve his or her own compensation). Nonetheless, the following remarks should be of interest to CEOs. If the CEO serves on the board, the CEO can urge the board to establish an effective, independent compensation committee that will in turn institute an effective process for recommending and approving executive pay. Furthermore, if the CEO also serves as chairman of the board (as sometimes occurs in diversified, for-profit healthcare concerns), the CEO can lead the creation of such a process—while at the same time remaining detached from its actual operation.

One source of guidance on the formation and operation of a compensation committee is the *Report of the NACD Blue Ribbon Commission on Executive Compensation* (1993/2000). This report is in essence a manifesto on executive compensation, signed by the 25 prominent individuals who drafted it. The individuals were a mix of compensation consultants, corporate executives, academicians, shareholder activists, and former regulators (two former members of the Securities and Exchange Commission).

The report outlines the following major compensation concerns of the directors and officers of any entity, including a healthcare organization:

- The role and composition of the compensation committee
- How much it should pay executives
- How it should pay executives
- How it should disclose those payments

The remainder of this chapter will focus on healthcare issues within these four subjects. All of these topics (plus others) are covered in greater depth later in this book.

THE ROLE OF THE CHAIRMAN OF THE BOARD IN SETTING COMPENSATION

The chairman of the board has a distinct job description, although it may not be written down as such. As a rule, most not-for-profit healthcare organizations separate the chairman and CEO. The two roles may be combined in the for-profit organization, and often are in larger, diversified healthcare concerns. In either case, it is important to distinguish the role of the chairman from the role of the CEO.

The chairman directs the board as it oversees the healthcare entity. The CEO, by contrast, manages the entity—with the support of key officers such as the president, chief operating officer (COO), chief financial officer (CFO), or treasurer. In hospitals, the medical staff president is a key officer.

Board Chairman's Position Description: Sample Elements

In directing the board, a chairman has a variety of duties. The following is a generic list of such duties, with annotations (in italics) that describe the chairman's specific role in setting executive compensation.[1]

The board chairman:

- Provides leadership to the board. *The chairman provides leadership to the board in developing, reviewing, and approving compensation policies.*
- Establishes procedures to govern the board's work (or, if also serving as the CEO, abides by such procedures as set by outside directors). *Establishes procedures to govern the work of the board in relation to compensation.*
- Ensures the board's full discharge of its duties. *Ensures the discharge of board duties related to compensation.*
- Schedules meetings of the full board and works with committee chairmen to coordinate the schedule of meetings for committees. *Works with the compensation committee chairman to ensure scheduling of compensation committee meetings.*
- Organizes and presents the agenda for regular or special board meetings based on input from directors. *Includes key compensation issues in the agenda for regular or special board meetings, as needed.*
- Ensures proper flow of information to the board, reviewing adequacy and timing of documentary materials in support of management's proposals. *Ensures proper flow of compensation information to the compensation committee of the board, reviewing adequacy and timing of materials.*
- Ensures adequate lead time for effective study and discussion of business under consideration. *Ensures adequate lead time for effective study and discussion of compensation matters under consideration.*
- Oversees the preparation and distribution of proxy materials to shareholders. *Ensures that proxy materials include necessary disclosures on executive compensation. If chairman of a not-for-profit, oversees the preparation and distribution of reports to regulators, contributors, and others.*
- Helps the board fulfill the goals it sets by assigning specific tasks to members of the board. *Helps the board fulfill the compensation policies and goals it sets by assigning specific tasks to the*

compensation committee of the board, or other board members as needed.

- Identifies guidelines for the conduct of the directors, and ensures that each director is making a significant contribution. *Ensures that guidelines for director conduct and contributions are linked to director compensation.*
- Acts as liaison between the board and management. (If also serving as CEO, delegates this duty to a lead director). *Serves as liaison between the board and management in the development, review, and approval of compensation policies.*
- Together with the CEO, represents the company to external groups such as sponsors, shareholders, creditors, consumer groups, local communities, and federal, state, and local governments. *Together with the CEO, represents the company with respect to compensation issues. Serves as lead representative, with the compensation committee chairman, on the subject of CEO compensation.*
- Works with the nominating committee to ensure proper committee structure, including assignments of members and committee chairmen. *Ensures the appointment of an independent, qualified individual and compensation committee chairman, and ensures appropriate rotation of this role.*
- Carries out other duties as requested by the CEO and board as a whole, depending on need and circumstances. *Accepts assignments related to compensation policy, as needed.*

The CEO's Position Description: Sample Elements

The CEO of a healthcare organization:

- Fosters an [organizational] culture that promotes ethical practices, encourages individual integrity, and fulfills social responsibility. *The CEO opposes policies that would confuse corporate ethics, weaken individual integrity, or violate the letter or spirit of any relevant laws or regulations.*

- Maintains a positive and ethical work climate that is conducive to attracting, retaining, and motivating a diverse group of top-quality employees at all levels. *The CEO implements compensation policies that attract, motivate, and reward excellence.*

- Develops and recommends to the board a long-term strategy and vision for the [organization]. *The CEO helps the board chairman and compensation committee link compensation to the organization's strategy and vision.*

- Develops and recommends to the board annual business plans and budgets that support the company's long-term strategy. *In presenting plans and budgets to the board, includes compensation plans and budgets that support the company's long-term strategy.*

- Ensures that the day-to-day business affairs of the company are appropriately managed. *Ensures that compensation plans are appropriately managed.*

- Consistently strives to achieve the [organization's] financial and operating goals and objectives. *Consistently strives to achieve all the organization's financial and operating goals and objectives, not only the ones expressed in the CEO's incentive arrangements.*

- Ensures continuous improvement in the quality and value of the products and services provided by the [organization]. *Encourages a link between compensation and quality, both with respect to his or her own pay, and the pay of others.*

- Ensures that the [organization] achieves and maintains a satisfactory competitive position within its industry. *Encourages a link between compensation and competitive position, both with respect to his or her own pay, and the pay of others.*

- Ensures that the company has an effective management team below the level of the CEO, and has an active plan in place for the CEO position. *Makes sure that compensation plans support succession plans.*

- Formulates and oversees the implementation of major [organizational] policies. *Formulates and oversees the implementation of compensation policies.*
- Serves as chief spokesperson for the [organization]. *Represents the organization with respect to compensation issues, sharing that role with the chairman of the board and the chairman of the compensation committee as appropriate.*

THE ROLE OF THE COMPENSATION COMMITTEE

"The compensation committee of the board of directors plays a critical role in *overseeing the compensation plans* for the [organization's] top executives, and often for directors as well. The members of that committee *forge the key link for the board and management* in balancing the interests of shareholders with those of management" (NACD 1993/2000).

This opening statement of the *Report of the NACD Blue Ribbon Commission on Executive Compensation* captures the main role of the board in a for-profit healthcare institution. It also sets an important standard for the not-for-profit institution, substituting the word "beneficiaries," or, more broadly, "stakeholders," for the word "shareholders."

The question, though, is this. How, precisely, can the board of directors (or trustees) oversee compensation plans—both as a full board and through a compensation committee? In assessing the effectiveness of a compensation plan, what should they look for? The Commission points out that committees need to do two things:

1. Review past [organizational] performance.
2. Compare past, current, and planned CEO and senior executive pay in relation to performance.

There are many measures of "performance." For all entities, this certainly includes financial performance as measured by financial statements. Patterns in revenues, profits, and key ratios all indicate performance. For the publicly held corporation, stock price is an obvious performance indicator—one, in fact, synonymous with shareholder wealth. In a not-for-profit entity, it is good, but not essential, to be profitable—or, in the language of the not-for-profit, to have "excess over expenses." The true imperative is to advance the mission of the entity.

Consider the mission of one Roman Catholic hospital located in the northeastern United States. It seeks to "provide a broad continuum of care, responding to the evolving needs of our...community." Striving to be "available to all persons," the hospital is devoted to "enhancing the quality of life at all stages, promoting health of body, mind, and spirit."

Furthermore, the mission statement declares that the hospital "integrates mission with sound business decisions."

In evaluating the performance of the CEO of this hospital, a chairman and a compensation committee would take these elements into account. The compensation committee of such a hospital would want assurance that, in addition to meeting any targets for revenue growth or sound financial performance, the hospital provided physical, mental, and spiritual service to all persons who need it. Compensation incentives might be based on particular aspects of this mission that seem weaker than others—a particular kind of service (e.g., mental health) to a particular group (e.g., the elderly).

In addition to looking at their own mission statements, healthcare organizations can consider the performance standards set forth in the 1993 report of the American College of Healthcare Executives, *Evaluating the Performance of the Hospital CEO in a Total Quality Management Environment*. ACHE established three important categories for top executive leadership ability and performance accountability:

1. Area-wide health status (e.g., community healthcare, social services projects)
2. Institutional success (e.g., human resource management, quality management, regulatory compliance, and advocacy).
3. Professional role fulfillment (e.g., continuing education, involvement in the profession).

As this report and Chapter 3 of this book reveal, performance evaluation of senior executives is a many-faceted activity. It cannot possibly be accomplished by a group of individuals who convene only once a month or every other month. However, these individuals can ensure that a proper process does exist, can independently monitor that process, and use its results to approve compensation packages.[2]

In awarding pay, compensation committee members should be sensitive to pay levels—that is, the actual amount of pay awarded. For-profit institutions have no restrictions on the level of pay, but shareholders do pay attention to it. In the past few years, institutional shareholders have filed a number of proxy resolutions and published attacks on high executive pay, including pay awarded at a major healthcare institution (Columbia/HCA).

For example, a major institutional investor, The American Federation of Labor–Congress of Industrial Organizations (AFL-CIO) posts examples of excessive CEO pay on its web site (www.afl-cio.org/paywatch). Also, a web-based information service for institutional investors, The Corporate Library (at www.thecorporatelibrary.com), publishes the full text of CEO pay agreements in public companies, and comments on excesses. The web site was founded by a past president of Institutional Shareholder Services, Inc. (www.iss.com), a well-known shareholder advisory firm. Several such web sites exist, providing ample materials to a media eager to report on excesses (see Chapter 9). With such obvious shareholder interest in pay levels, compensation committees of for-profit institutions must be absolutely certain to link pay to performance and avoid overly generous pay.

Not-for-profit institutions have definite restrictions on pay levels under U. S. tax law. As discussed in Chapter 4, in 1996 Congress enacted legislation that can affect the compensation arrangements between not-for-profit organizations and certain individuals. Not-for-profit directors should review their organization's compensation arrangements in light of IRC Section 4958, or what is commonly referred to as *intermediate sanctions*. Directors of nontaxable organizations must disclose excessive compensation on Form 990 (discussed in Chapter 4 and at the end of this chapter).

THE ROLE OF THE CHAIRMAN OF THE COMPENSATION COMMITTEE

All board committees need an effective chairman—a man or woman who will convene the committee, set the agenda, bring out full and candid discussion of the issues facing the committee, and propose actions to the full board of directors. The chairman of the compensation committee has an intensified duty in this regard. As mentioned earlier, the compensation committee should be entirely independent of the healthcare entity. Therefore, the chairman—who is also independent of the organization— must develop the relationships with the necessary professionals to obtain the information needed to fulfill the committee's responsibilities.

Compensation Committee Chairman's Position Description: Sample Elements

The following is a sample position description of the chairman of a compensation committee, as provided in *The Compensation Committee Manual* (Richard 1999).

Basic Function:

Presides at all meetings of the committee. Presents findings and recommendations to the board in reviewing and deciding upon matters that exert major influence on the manner in which the organization's executives are paid. Performs such duties as may be conferred by law or assigned by the full board.

Responsibilities:

- Prepares agenda for and convenes and conducts regular and special meetings of the committee.
- Advises and gives counsel to other board members of the organization.
- Reviews major activities and plans to ensure conformity with the board's views on corporate compensation and policy.
- Carries out such special assignments.
- Counsels collectively and individually with members of the board, utilizing their capacities to the fullest extent necessary to secure optimum benefits for the corporation.
- May nominate directors for committee involvement.
- Presents any proposed changes in major policies of the corporation for board action.
- Retains and works with outside consultants when necessary.

The compensation committee should set forth these duties in a written charter. For a sample charter, see Figure 1.1.

COMPOSITION OF THE COMPENSATION COMMITTEE: STANDARDS FOR INDEPENDENCE

Whether directors are measuring CEO performance based on meeting a financial goal, a mission statement, or both, they need to

Figure 1.1: A Sample Compensation Committee Charter

The Compensation Committee

Purpose

To review and report to the board on compensation and personnel policies, programs, and plans, including management development and succession plans, and to approve employee compensation and benefit programs.

Membership

The compensation committee is composed entirely of outside directors.

Oversight Areas for Compensation Strategy

• Compensation policies and programs
• Compensation levels of directors, CEO, president, top officers, and management group (Full board must approve compensation policy with respect to directors, CEO, and president.)
• Succession planning
• Management development
• Compensation and employee benefit plans
• Administration of stock bonus plans, stock option plans, non-employee director stock plans, and other executive and director compensation arrangements

Agenda Items

The activities of the compensation committee are developed from year to year by the committee in consultation with management. The compensation committee typically meets three times a year.

February
• Long-term incentive compensation
• Restricted stock-plan awards
• Base salaries (executive officers)

July
• Grants of stock options

Figure 1.1 *(continued)*

November

- Top management bonuses
- Key employee compensation awards
- All-employee bonuses
- Policies and processes for development of employees
- Progress in compliance with labor laws
- Management resources available versus current needs
- Projected resources vs. current needs

Approve as needed:

- Changes in appointments
- Changes in compensation plans
- Changes in benefit plans

Source: National Association of Corporate Directors. 2000. *Board Policy Manual.* Washington, DC: NACD.

exercise objective judgment. It is generally believed that the best evaluation comes from disinterested, independent parties. As mentioned earlier, it is now widely believed that CEO pay should be set by a board compensation committee composed entirely of *independent* outside directors. The reason for this is obvious: an independent committee is more likely to be fair and impartial in awarding CEO pay. If any members work for the CEO, or provide services to the company, they may find it difficult to adopt an objective attitude toward the CEO's compensation.

No laws, regulations, or rules currently require the independent composition of compensation committees (although IRC Section 162(m) requires such composition for deducting pay over $1 million). However, the New York Stock Exchange and the American Stock Exchange require independent audit committees, defining independence very narrowly in their 1999 rules. Some governance experts believe that the exchanges will some day set forth a similar requirement for compensation committees.

Securities and tax laws extend certain regulatory exemptions for payments approved by independent directors. Consider for example the exceptions available under Rule 16(b)3 of the Securities Exchange Act of 1934, administered by the U.S. Securities and Exchange Commission. The 1934 Act's Rule 16(b), known as the "short-swing" rule, prohibits insiders from buying and selling the company's stock within a six-month period. Rule 16(b)3, as amended in 1996, provides an exemption for certain transactions involving stock-based awards, as long as the awards were approved by a committee composed solely of two or more "non-employee" directors.

Rule 16(b)3 defines a non-employee director broadly as a director who:

- is not currently an officer or otherwise employed by the issuer or a parent or subsidiary of the company.
- does not receive compensation, either directly or indirectly, from the company or a parent or subsidiary of the company, for services rendered as a consultant or in any capacity other than as a director, except for an amount that does not exceed the dollar amount for which disclosure would be required under Regulation S-K, Item 404(a). (This item requires disclosure of compensation exceeding $60,000.)
- is not engaged in a business relationship for which disclosure would be required under Regulation S-K, Item 404(b). (This item lists various types of business relationships, including employment in the company, a vendor to the company, or a law firm or bank providing services to the company.)

Another relevant exemption (and definition) is set forth by the Internal Revenue Service of the United States Treasury in relation to independent directors serving on compensation committees. This definition was issued in 1993 in relation to a new section of the Internal Revenue Code (IRC) Section 162(m).

IRC Section 162(m) sets a $1 million limit on the amount of executive pay that will be tax-deductible as an ordinary business expense. The only exception to this cap is performance-based pay awarded by a compensation committee composed solely of two or more independent outside directors.

Section 162(m) defines an independent director as one who:

- is not a current employee of the company or its affiliates.
- is not a former employee who receives compensation for prior services (other than from a tax-exempt retirement plan).
- is not a current or former officer.
- does not receive remuneration, directly or indirectly, in any capacity other than as a director.

The remuneration counts if it is received via an entity the director controls (having more than 50 percent beneficial interest). It also counts if it is paid to an entity that employs the director, or that the director owns as a minority shareholder (having between 5 and 50 percent). In the latter cases, however, the amount is exempt if it is $60,000 or less.

Shareholder groups also have guidelines for independence. For example, the Council for Institutional Investors (CII) has a definition, which was most recently expanded in March 2000. The CII definition is similar to the stock exchange, securities law, and tax law definitions explained above, but adds three extra characteristics. Members of the CII do not consider directors independent if they are current employees of or vendors to the company, if they worked for the company in the past two years. Furthermore, in *addition* to these requirements, the CII does not consider a director independent if he or she:

- is a relative of a company executive (a restriction that also appears in the New York Stock Exchange and Nasdaq requirements for audit committees, incidentally).
- is an employee, officer, or director of a foundation, university, or other not-for-profit organization that receives significant grants or endowments from the corporation or one of its affiliates.

- is part of an interlocking directorate in which the CEO or other executive officer of the corporation on the board of another corporation that employs the director.

Officers and directors of healthcare organizations seeking to create independent compensation committees are advised to establish their own guidelines, suited to their specific situations. If the organizations are private, there are no special regulatory or relational reasons to do so—but having an independence definition would be a sound policy (a simple definition based on 16(b)3 rules would suffice). If the organization is a public company, it would do well to use the 162(m) definition. If the organization has owners that are major institutional investors, the most stringent CII definition would be the best place to start. Not-for-profit organizations will do well by following the guidelines for independence set forth in Chapter 4 of this book (see the discussion on prohibitions against inurement in tax-exempt organizations).

Compensation Committee Membership and Activities

So far we have seen the role of the compensation committee and have learned that there are many regulatory advantages to composing this committee entirely of outsiders. Now the question is, how many members should it have and what exactly should it do?

Kesner et al. (1995) has noted that "over time, many compensation committees have grown and taken on added responsibilities without adapting their structures to suit changed conditions." In an article on compensation committees, they recommend that committees should be:

- large enough to ensure differing viewpoints.
- based on staggered tenures long enough to implement long-term strategies but short enough to ensure a regular infusion of new ideas and new perspectives.

- composed of three to five outside directors who can exercise sound judgment independent of top management.

Furthermore, Kesner suggests that boards should assign audit committee service to individuals who have a "basic understanding of compensation issues." Kesner also suggests that committees meet three or four times per year to deal with specific issues on a "well-planned, timely basis." Finally, he suggests that the committee set forth a charter that defines the committee's responsibilities, and lists all issues that need approval by the full board of directors.

These issues may include developing, reviewing, and monitoring the company's:

- executive compensation philosophy;
- executive compensation programs;
- executive performance measurements;
- allocation of annual bonuses to eligible executives;
- executive employment contracts;
- profit-sharing and benefit plans (although there may be a separate committee for this);
- the annual CEO performance review; and
- disclosure of compensation.

The compensation committee may also be responsible for setting director pay, but not usually for evaluating director performance. Increasingly, boards are using a governance or directors committee to lead the board in that exercise.

DISCLOSURE DUTIES OF THE COMPENSATION COMMITTEE

The board of directors has significant disclosure responsibilities with respect to executive compensation. In many cases, these duties are delegated to the compensation committee and its advisors.

Directors of healthcare institutions that are publicly traded must adhere to the SEC's disclosure rules. For many decades, the SEC required a great number of disclosures on compensation; however, there was no standard format for the disclosures, which made them difficult to understand. In 1992, the SEC passed detailed rules standardizing disclosures about the CEO and the four other most highly compensated individuals (whose annual salary exceeds $100,000).

Under Regulation S-K, public companies must disclose the following information for these most highly paid individuals:

- A summary table containing detailed information and total compensation, disclosing three years base salary, bonuses, long-term compensation, and all other forms of cash and non-cash compensation awarded
- Tables showing options or stock appreciation rights that show potential appreciation on newly granted options, actual appreciation realized on exercised options, and unrealized gain on outstanding options (both exercisable and unexercisable)

Public companies must also prepare and disclose a performance graph comparing the company's five-year shareholder returns with those of other companies, using both a broad market index and an industry index.

In addition to showing these three charts, companies must also disclose the following:

- Policies governing executive compensation
- Relationship between the company's performance and the compensation to these most highly paid executives
- The basis for the CEO's pay the previous year
- Criteria for the CEO's current pay
- The relationship between the CEO's performance and that of the company

- Each measure the committee used to set the CEO's compensation, whether qualitative or quantitative

Furthermore, the boards of not-for-profit healthcare institutions have disclosure responsibilities. As explained in Chapter 4, a not-for-profit organization has a reporting responsibility with regard to intermediate sanctions. If an excess benefit transaction occurs, the organization discloses this on its annual Form 990, *Return of Organization Exempt from Income Tax*. Form 990, which is open to the public, requires the organization to describe the type of transaction, identify the person involved, and state whether the transaction was corrected. Form 990 filers must also disclose the amount of intermediate sanctions tax, if any, paid by the person.

CONCLUSION

The compensation committees of healthcare organizations clearly have a great deal of important work to do. The following chapters are dedicated not only to compensation committee members, but also to their director and officer colleagues, including the chairman and CEO. This material can help healthcare leaders master all the most important issues in healthcare compensation today.

NOTES

1. This list is reprinted with permission from the *Report of the NACD Blue Ribbon Commission on Director Professionalism* (Washington, DC: National Association of Corporate Directors), p. 35. In this chapter, it includes compensation-related annotations from the author (Thomas P. Flannery).

2. Chapter 3 of *Evaluating the Performance of the Hospital CEO in a Total Quality Management Environment* (ACHE 1993) focuses on the process of evaluating the performance of a hospital CEO

including eight guidelines as to who should evaluate the CEO and how often this should take place, as well as the issue of tying the CEO's compensation to his/her performance. An appendix sets forth guidelines for evaluation of the CEO based on a review of accountabilities of CEOs.

REFERENCES

American College of Healthcare Executives. 1993. *Evaluating the Performance of the Hospital CEO in a Total Quality Management Environment*. Chicago: ACHE.

American College of Healthcare Executives, American Hospital Association, American Medical Association, and Ernst & Young. 1993. *The Partnership Study: A Study of the Roles and Working Relationships of the Hospital Board Chairman, CEO, and Medical Staff President; Survey Findings*. Chicago: ACHE.

Kesner, M., F. A. Rossi, and P. Lapides. 1995. "Guidelines for More Effective Compensation Committees." *Director's Monthly* (August) 7–10.

National Association of Corporate Directors (NACD). 1993/2000. *The Report of the NACD Blue Ribbon Commission on Executive Compensation: Guidelines for Corporate Directors* Washington, DC: NACD.

National Association of Corporate Directors (NACD). 2000. *Board Policy Manual*. Washington, DC: NACD.

Richard, J. E. 1999. *Compensation Committee Manual*, 4th ed. Half Moon Bay, CA: J. E. Richard & Co.

CHAPTER 2

Compensation Elements and Trends

Thomas P. Flannery and Deborah L. Rose

AS ESTABLISHED IN Chapter 1, healthcare board members have an important role in setting and implementing executive pay policy. Furthermore, executives themselves, whether serving on the board or not, must address their own compensation. This chapter will provide information and approaches that directors, officers, and other senior executives can use to understand and master the dynamics of compensation in the broader context of governing and managing a successful healthcare organization.

Because there is nothing terribly complex about the concepts of base salary, bonuses, and the like, some of the information in this chapter may seem basic. However, in today's highly accountable compensation environment—with shareholders, executives, and regulators all favoring pay for performance—the elements themselves are not what really matter. Rather, what counts most is the interaction of the elements as part of the entire reward relationship between the healthcare institution and its key executives.

TOTAL REMUNERATION DEFINED

Understanding executive compensation dynamics begins with an understanding of "total remuneration," also called "total rewards." We use this term to describe the financial portion of the relationship between the executive and the organization. It is the value of all parts of the executive compensation package, which is divided into four key parts.

1. Cash compensation consists of three main parts:
    *   *Base salary* is the regular payment provided to the executive for the performance of services. It reflects what the board is willing to pay for expected performance. Base salary at the executive level is defined in terms of annual pay.
    *   *Incentive compensation* is designed to reward for performance above expected levels. It is usually defined as short-term or long-term compensation. Short-term incentives are usually for performance of one year or less and long-term incentives are usually for performance of two or more years.
    *   *Bonus compensation* is a payment for meritorious services "after-the-fact." It is usually a discretionary payment, unlike an incentive plan that rewards for achievement of specified performance goals. It is unusual for an executive to receive both an incentive and a bonus payment. (Note: payments commonly called "signing bonuses" and "retention bonuses" are not true bonus compensation in this sense).
2. Benefits are compensation elements (usually packaged together in the form of programs) designed to address specific employee needs. Within executive benefits programs are such elements as:
    *   *Health and welfare programs* that offer healthcare insurance (and sometimes other healthcare programs) for the executive and his or her family, salary continuation in the

event that the executive becomes disabled, and life insurance in case of the death of the executive.

- *Retirement programs,* which can be of two types, the broad-based kind and the "executive" kind. In the broad-based program, the executive participates in the organization's normal retirement program, which may be a traditional defined benefit program or a more contemporary defined contribution program. The second type of program is an executive retirement program. This type of program recognizes the unique retirement pay problems faced by an executive, such as the loss or reduction of retirement benefits because of changing jobs (often the case for a high-level executive recruited in mid-career), and the statutory limitations on executive retirement benefits. An executive retirement program offers additional retirement income to compensate for these problems.

- *Severance and other special pay programs* that frequently appear in contracts between healthcare organizations and their senior executives. As discussed in Chapter 6, this benefit suits the purposes of tax-exempt health systems and their employees because, if properly structured, it can qualify as a bona fide severance pay plan under Section 457, which contains an exception for such plans. This category also encompasses any special financial arrangements made as part of an employment contract, such as a signing or retention bonus (which, as mentioned, is not technically a true merit bonus).

- *Time-off programs* that include vacation, holiday, and sick leave. The trend today is to provide "paid-time-off" programs where the executive (or other employee), is given a fixed number of days without stipulating how the time is to be allocated between vacation, holidays, and/or sick leave.

3. Equity compensation rewards executives (or other employees) for contributing to the financial success of a healthcare

business by allowing the executive to participate in some version of a stock program. Equity compensation can be paid in the form of outright stock grants or in the form of options to buy stock in the future at certain predetermined prices. Stock grants may be simple grants, or they may be restricted to a particular time period to encourage the executive to stay with the organization. In some cases, rather than being awarded the stock, executives are required or encouraged to buy the stock as part of an organization's stock ownership policy (for example, some boards require executives to adhere to stock ownership guidelines). Although equity compensation is most typically found in publicly held companies, it can also be found in privately held companies, partnerships, and not-for-profit organizations, which use "phantom share" programs. Phantom share programs will be discussed as a long-term incentive program later in this chapter.

4. Perquisites, nicknamed "perks," are the supplemental elements in the compensation program. These extras may include automobiles, club memberships, financial counseling, or supplemental life, medical, or disability insurance. Because they are not usually connected to performance, and can be viewed as excessive, perquisites are gradually losing favor. They are being replaced through additions to the executive's base salary or, in more progressive organizations, additions to equity compensation.

Each of these elements should be valued and disclosed. If the organization is publicly held, it must make certain disclosures in its proxy 10-K, and other financial reports under Regulation S-K, as described in Chapter 1. If it is a not-for-profit institution, it must make disclosures on its Form 990 to demonstrate that it is not awarding "excessive" compensation to its key employees. (For more on Regulation S-K, see Chapter 1. For more on Form 990 and the related topic of intermediate sanctions, see Chapter 4.)

Valuing cash compensation and cash-based perquisites is a straightforward matter. Cash compensation is simply the actual amount of cash paid out (in whatever form) during the fiscal year. Time-off programs require valuing and reporting only if paid in cash in lieu of the executive taking the time off.

The more difficult tasks lie in valuing certain kinds of equity-based compensation and certain benefit programs. Equity-based compensation, as mentioned, may be awarded as grants of stock or options. Stock grants can be easily valued by multiplying the amount of stock awarded times the price of the stock at the time of the award. Valuing unexercised stock options is more complex. Although several ways exist to do this, the Securities and Exchange Commission, in Regulation S-K, details specific requirements. It requires organizations to report, in chart form, the number of options granted to the CEO and the four highest-paid executives; the percentage of total options granted to each executive; the exercise price of the stock options; the expiration date; and the "potential realizable value at assumed annual rates of stock price appreciation for the option term, assuming 5 percent and 10 percent growth scenarios, using the actual option term and accrual compounding." Regulation S-K also requires certain additional disclosures, such as "any standard or formula that may adjust exercise or base price."

Benefit programs are similarly complex when it comes to valuation. There are basically two ways to value benefit programs. The simplest way is to use the actual cost of the program, as paid by the organization for the benefit of the executive. There is also a "common cost" methodology that adjusts the value of the benefit so as to normalize the cost across different population groups.

Specific benefit programs such as split-dollar life insurance are particularly difficult to value. As described in Chapter 5, many kinds of split-dollar programs exist, and the Internal Revenue Service (IRS) is in the process of changing its rules regarding the valuation of these benefits. (The IRS looks at these issues on an ongoing basis.) Another complex question is whether organizations need to disclose the potential value of future income under executive employment contracts, such as retention bonuses or change of control provisions (known as "golden parachutes") payable at a future date. Organizations should retain expert compensation consulting advisors to work with their legal advisors on such matters.

CRITERIA FOR SETTING TOTAL REWARD

Setting total rewards for top executives requires leadership from the board of directors. They must oversee and approve the development of compensation packages that the organization is both *willing* and *able* to pay, given the strategic and practical issues it faces.

Following are some of the strategic issues (questions) that a board must consider.

- What are the healthcare objectives of the organization? Is the organization changing its care pattern in any significant way?
- Where is the organization in its life cycle—growth, stability, decline, or renewal through restructuring?
- What are the most critical issues facing the organization, and are they short- or long-term issues? Does the board anticipate needing a specialist to "turn around" the organization? What specialized skills will be required—clinical, financial, human resources? During what period of time will these skills be required?
- Where does the organization stand with respect to consolidation and alliances in the industry—is it buying companies, selling subsidiaries, and/or contemplating a major merger? What about joint ventures or other strategic alliances?
- What level of risk is the organization facing (not only financial but also in terms of quality, reputation, and employee, community, and physician relations)? Do directors and officers understand these risks? Do they have the competencies required to mitigate them?

- Has there been significant turnover in the executive ranks? What is the cause of the turnover? Is it related to relationship issues involving the board versus senior management, or senior management versus key employees, such as physicians? How can these relationships improve?
- Does the organization have any challenges with respect to its reputation, or legacy issues? Have the legacy issues spilled into the public arena? If so, how will these issues affect the ability of the organization to attract quality candidates? (For more on reputation management, see Chapter 9.)

Considering these strategic issues can bring perspective to decision makers (typically members of the board's compensation committee) and to the organization's compensation advisors. Understanding these issues brings better insight into how to link the compensation strategy to the business strategy. A well-designed compensation plan will motivate the behaviors necessary to accomplish the business strategy of the organization.

These issues are very important to executive recruitment. By discussing these high-level issues with senior executive candidates, organization leaders can make sure the candidates are prepared for the challenges ahead. For these reasons, as one board member of a for-profit healthcare company has commented, directors must put these issues "squarely on the table" when hiring a chief executive officer. The CEO, in turn, must also put these issues on the table when employing members of the executive team.

In addition to these strategic issues, several important practical issues can help decision makers set policies for CEO and executive pay.

- The candidate's experience and talents obviously play a role. Some organizations need candidates with specific experience in government, technology, managed care, or other fields. Other organizations may need specific talents, such as an ability to serve as liaison between groups in conflict. In the decision to hire and compensate a candidate, factors like these need to be considered. This is especially true if the candidate is the only one with similar experience or talents, and if the experience or talent sought mitigates a critical risk factor.

- Availability of similar talent adds another dimension—especially if the search must be limited geographically (as it often must be, since few candidates want to relocate). In the healthcare industry today, the demand for excellent executive talent exceeds the supply. Given the specific experience and talents the organization needs, there may not be a great deal of choice about whether a candidate should be hired; the only question will be for how much.

- The candidate's current level of compensation is the obvious starting point. In changing jobs—especially if this calls for a geographic move that will uproot the candidate and the candidate's family—most people will have a minimum compensation threshold they will accept. Generally, we see this minimum as a 15 to 20 percent increase if the change is for the same role at a similar institution.

- Compensation market data (in order to benchmark or emulate what other organizations are paying for similar work) also merits consideration in most cases. Compensation survey information can always be helpful. It is especially relevant when the candidate is expected to move to a new area (especially one with a higher cost of living) or assume a role with greater scope, size, or accountability (whether or not this increase is reflected in the new title).

COMPENSATION MARKET DATA

Given the importance of compensation market data, it is clearly worthwhile for organizations to gather market data before awarding pay. There are different types of surveys, some of which are more valuable than others. When assessing the usefulness of a survey, decision makers should consider the following.

- *Representativeness of the market.* Does the survey reflect the market(s) from which you will recruit or lose talent? For example, if rural hospitals dominate the survey, it will probably not be useful for organizations in major urban areas.
- *Range of positions.* Does the survey include most, if not all, of the executive positions in your organization?
- *Compensation elements.* Are all of the elements of compensation included in the survey? Many surveys do not include, or have limited information about, some of the most important elements, such as benefit programs.
- *Data cuts.* Does the survey provider allow you to make specific comparisons between your organization and a segment of the participants in the survey? This will help you to narrow the comparisons to better reflect the market within which you compete for talent.
- *Trends.* Is there information about current executive compensation trends, including explanations about year-to-year changes in levels or design of compensation?
- *Methodology.* Does the survey explain how researchers collected the data? As explained more fully below, methodologies vary, and some are more valid than others.

Elaborating further on the subject of methodology, there are several types of surveys.

- *Club surveys.* A club survey yields the best information, assuming that it reflects the issues described above. It is called a club survey because participants have some affiliation, such as belonging to the same trade association. If the American College of Healthcare Executives were to select a random sample of members, and survey these same members year after year, this would be an example of a club survey. As this example indicates, the source of the affiliation (such as an association) is typically the sponsor of the survey. This is generally a survey of organizations that are similar in demographic factors, such as its industry sector, geographic market, size, scope, and reputation. Only participants may see the results of the survey. Participants usually agree to participate in the survey each year and share the data for setting executive compensation. This type of survey is very beneficial because it offers high quality, consistent responses over time, since the same respondents answer year after year. The downside is often the cost of the survey, both in collecting the data and completing data submission kits (remember, only participants receive results).

- *Filing-based surveys.* Some compensation surveys are based on publicly available information. Publicly traded companies are required to file annual proxy statements that include compensation information. Not-for-profit organizations file IRS Form 990, which also contains compensation information. These documents can be used to cull data. The benefit of these databases is that fairly high quality data is obtained; the downside is that the information may not be timely or complete.

- *General surveys.* These are surveys of a large population, not just members of a specific group. In this kind of survey, the researchers send the survey questionnaire to a large number of organizations, which may or may not choose to participate. The sponsors of these surveys are usually trade, academic, or consulting organizations that have a profession, scholarly, or commercial use for the data, so they do not charge very much for the survey results—and may even publish them for free. The benefit of this survey is that the cost of purchase is fairly modest; the downside is that the survey responses may be biased, because survey respondents are not selected randomly, but select themselves. Therefore, they may not be representative of the entire population.

Two additional survey types warrant an examination. These surveys have value, but should be used in combination with at least one of the above kinds of surveys, since their applicability may be limited.

- *Periodical surveys.* Two quality magazines, *Modern Healthcare* and *Health and Hospitals Network,* among others, publish executive compensation data. The data reported in such periodicals are gathered using sound methods (club, filing-based, or general). However, the positions featured in the magazines are not always comparable to the positions in your organization, because they tend to report only a few executive positions for an average institution, rather than reporting several senior positions by a variety of organizational sizes, types, locations, etc. While the issues on executive compensation are probably the best-read ones these magazines produce, decision makers should use them only in conjunction with other published data sources.
- *Trade surveys.* A number of trade organizations publish compensation information for specific job functions, such as materials management or information technology. These surveys, published quite frequently (sometimes quarterly) are good for a specific position, but should only be used in concert with other data sources.

Having worked with all these kinds of surveys, we recommend that pay decision makers do the following:

- Participate in at least one club survey.
- Include at least two additional general surveys from quality providers.
- Secure additional data if the board has any question about the quality of the surveys.

Each survey that you use should:

- Cover positions equal or similar to those on your executive team.
- Contain all elements of compensation (cash, benefits, equity compensation, perquisites).
- Cover your geographic market or one with a comparable cost of living.
- Cover organizations of similar size and scope.
- Cover organizations in your industry segment (for example, hospitals, home healthcare providers, and health insurers are three different healthcare sectors).

If no single survey fills all these requirements, you can use multiple surveys to piece together a picture. For example, one survey might cover cash compensation in the CEO position and another survey might cover cash compensation in the CFO position. Yet another survey might cover benefits paid to the CEO and CFO. This can provide a very general idea; however, for true comparability, it is much better to have all the information come from the same survey.

Andersen LLP recently studied 990 forms to discern trends in healthcare compensation (see Appendix 2A). This type of information can be useful to many healthcare organizations. Often, healthcare organizations compare their compensation to their competitors using the IRS 990 Form information. The market competitor group should be composed of the healthcare organizations most similar to the healthcare organization conducting the analysis. Common criteria for the market competitor group are business strategy, size of healthcare organization, number of beds, for-profit, not-for-profit, academic, and/or non-academic. Where IRS 990 Form data is insufficient, the healthcare organization may either broaden the competitor group or supplement the IRS 990 Form data with other compensation survey data. Compensation reported in the 990 Form is, most commonly, base salary and annual incentive paid.

Relying exclusively on surveys, however, can pose a number of problems.

- Surveys rarely report the highest and lowest paid incumbent for a particular position. A survey may report, for example, the 10th through 90th percentile but not compensation practices below or above those levels. This leaves out information that may be important to organizations that pay very low or very high amounts (e.g., in the 5th or 95th percentile).
- It is virtually impossible to track compensation elements in a consistent manner. For example, a survey may report cash compensation on 100 chief operating officers (COOs), but it may not distinguish between those who received the cash in the form of both base salary and incentives, versus those who received base salary *only* for that particular year. This means that unless decision makers are very careful, they may draw the wrong conclusions from the data.
- Some compensation elements (especially benefits and perquisites) are reported in terms of prevalence—that is, the percentage of survey participants that offer the element. This is interesting, but the surveys usually do not indicate what positions receive the compensation element. For example, a survey may report that 75 percent of all participating organizations provide supplemental life insurance, but make no mention of the fact that only the CEO receives this element.
- Over time, the number of organizations that provide a specific compensation element may decrease. Two decades ago a company car was common, while today fewer organizations provide this perquisite. Yet surveys rarely report that some organizations may have eliminated a car or car allowance and rolled an equivalent amount into the cash compensation program. A misreading of the survey may cause an organization (wanting to benchmark from the survey results) to raise its base salaries while also providing an automobile.

- It may be virtually impossible to find specific information such as the severance period in an employment contract or separation agreement.

Given the growing interest in the accurate reporting of executive compensation in both the for-profit and not-for-profit sectors, we expect that the quality of surveys will improve. For one thing, there is a growing trend to use online survey forms, which can increase response rates and improve timeliness (Meyer 2001). We foresee survey providers improving their methodology at the request of boards and CEOs. One key will be healthcare leaders themselves. One of the biggest barriers to accurate healthcare compensation surveys is the reluctance of healthcare organizations to take the time, effort, and care required to complete survey forms.

Better yet, decision makers can seek customized information and advice to supplement survey information. Surveys—except, perhaps, for customized club surveys—will not provide information in a way that provides solid comfort. This is why most boards use executive compensation consultants to help them through the compensation process.

TAXATION OF COMPENSATION ELEMENTS

Even assuming that an organization can obtain complete and accurate benchmark information about compensation levels, it needs to factor in its own unique circumstances. One very important circumstance to consider is the organization's tax situation. Whether the organization is a tax-exempt not-for-profit or a tax-paying, for-profit organization, it should be aware of current federal tax policies.

Generally, the federal approach to taxation is to tax everything that can be taxed—but how regulators do this is constantly changing. Decision makers, and those who are actually designing pay plans, should be aware of current tax regulations and rules and how they affect executive compensation programs. Again, engaging the services of a compensation specialist is recommended.

Automobiles provide an instructive example of the changing nature of pay taxation. Not too many years ago, it was possible to provide an automobile, virtually tax free, as a perquisite to the executive. Now this is virtually impossible. Today, if the vehicle is used more than 50 percent for personal use, it is fully taxable. Furthermore, two additional factors must be considered. First, if the executive commutes between home and work, this is considered personal use. This makes it very difficult to get the 50 percent business use that is required. Second, the executive has to keep records to substantiate the allocation between business and personal uses. Unless there are clear records—detailing date, mileage, purpose of the trip, and associated costs—the executive may not be able to substantiate the business purpose of the trip.

Given the federal government's attitude toward luxury cars and other questionable perquisites, healthcare organizations have shied away from perks, opting instead to increase cash compensation. This way, they stay out of the automobile buying or leasing business, their executives can buy or lease automobiles to reflect their personal tastes, and the IRS gets its tax payment.

Note, however, that although regulators take no particular note of automobiles purchased with a taxpayer's own money, the news media may criticize such purchases if they seem incongruous with the purpose of a not-for-profit organization. Fairly or unfairly, leaders of not-for-profits can expect public criticism if they drive luxury cars or own other items associated with conspicuous wealth.

POINTS OF COMPARISON

In any event, the decision to provide a benefit (e.g. health insurance, life insurance, or disability insurance) or perquisite (e.g. tuition reimbursement, club membership, supplemental life insurance, financial counseling, or child care) should be made with due comparison to other standards. It is best if decision makers can consider the benefit or perquisite to be a practice that fits an organizational practice, a competitive practice, or a useful practice, described as follows.

- *Organization practice.* Has the organization traditionally provided the benefit or the perquisite?
- *Competitive practice.* Is the benefit or perquisite normally provided to executives in other healthcare organizations? For example, it is standard to provide an employment contract for the CEO, include a "pension restoration plan" for those compensated over limits defined by pension law, and offer a voluntary deferred compensation program. In addition, spouse travel to support the executive in his or her business activities is often reimbursed.
- *Useful practice.* Some organizations offer special benefits and perquisites because they are useful in bringing about positive results. For example, for long-tenured executives, some organizations are now providing sabbaticals to maintain the executive's work-life balance. Having the use of a company-owned aircraft may also be useful. Although it is an unusual practice, some healthcare organizations justify this as a business necessity given the difficulty of travel to many of the facilities owned or operated by the organization.

In all cases, the board should have a clear business purpose to support the practice. Standard practices can be easily explained as a normal part of the relationship between the organization and all of its employees. Competitive practices should be supported with clear evidence as to the competitive nature of the benefit or perquisite. Useful practices should demonstrate the advantage that they will provide to the organization. For example, it is a better business practice to provide a two- or three-month sabbatical than to suffer the cost of recruitment fees and the instability caused by having to replace a CEO. Any unusual practices should be clearly documented as to the business purpose and the costs and benefits of the practice to the organization.

If a benefit or perquisite has no precedence in the organization or in the industry, and serves no useful purpose, it should be carefully assessed in light of the potential negative publicity that it may attract.

INCENTIVE PLANS AND PERFORMANCE MEASURES

Most healthcare organizations position base salary at competitive levels, such as the average or median of their competitive market. In addition, it is very common for healthcare organizations to have some type of annual incentive program for their executives—and sometimes for all managers within the organization. Annual incentive plans typically focus on goals that are achieved in 12 months or less. Many types of annual incentive plans exist. Some of the more common types include an annual bonus based on overall organization performance, an annual bonus based on individual performance against predetermined goals, and team incentives.

As discussed in Chapter 3, healthcare organizations typically use a mix of performance measures, weighted based on the organization's strategic objectives and goals. These performance measures may be financial or nonfinancial. Financial measures commonly used in incentive plans include gross margin, operating margin, and revenue growth. Nonfinancial measures commonly include patient satisfaction, employee satisfaction, and quality measures (including critical measures such as mortality rates). In addition, some incentive plans are based on individual performance, with targets based on doing better than before in specific areas.

Once the healthcare organization designs an annual incentive plan, each participant typically has a target bonus. The target bonus as a percentage of base salary varies greatly among healthcare organizations. At the executive level the target bonus amount can range from 20 to 75 percent of base salary. The actual payout of the target bonus amount typically ranges from 80 to 120 percent of the individual's target bonus. The actual payout is generally directly related to the performance of the healthcare organization and/or the individual, with more weight given to organizational performance for more senior executives.

Long-term incentive plans are much less common in the healthcare industry, but some healthcare organizations do have equity and/or cash based incentive plans. Typically, these plans focus on goals that span a period longer than 12 months.

COMPENSATION STRATEGY: A FEW KEY QUESTIONS

Determining the optimal cash compensation "mix" (i.e., proportion of base salary versus annual incentive versus long-term incentive) plays an important role in the overall strategy. The optimal mix is unique to each organization.

Compensation decision makers—typically members of the compensation committee of the board—should consider a broad range of questions when reviewing the organization's compensation strategy. The answer to these questions will help to design a total compensation system that complements the organization's business objectives and motivates all employees. Here are just a few of the questions to consider.

- Are executives' salaries and incentive opportunities competitive with the market?
- At what level should executives' salaries be positioned in the market? At market or slightly above or below market?
- Should we set limits on incentive pay?
- How should employees below the executive level be paid? Are cash incentives appropriate?

- What performance measures should be used in the incentive plan?
- Should incentives be based on overall financial measures or other measures such as market share and customer satisfaction?
- Should performance measures for employees be the same as for top executives?
- How often should incentives be paid?
- Should there be a minimum level of corporate performance before incentives are paid?
- Should we have a long-term incentive plan?
- Who should receive options, and how many?
- What percentage of equity should be reserved for executives and employees? Will there be enough for future hires and subsequent annual grants?
- Does a broad-based equity plan make sense?
- What specific provisions should be included in an equity plan (e.g., vesting schedules, change-in-control provisions)?

CONCLUSION

To be effective, the men and women entrusted with executive compensation decisions need information, strategy, and a broad understanding of the compensation process. They require information on compensation trends, practices, and levels—and must also understand the strategic implications of what they include in the compensation package. Finally, they must understand how the main elements of compensation interrelate. A solid foundation based on these elements can make compensation systems in health-care organizations more effective in recruiting, motivating, and retaining the best executives.

REFERENCE

Meyer, B. 2001. "Internet Surveys: From Data to Information and Back." *Human Capital*. New York: Profile Pursuit/Andersen.

Trends in Benefits and Perquisites: An Andersen Survey

The most recent *Andersen Survey of Health and Welfare Benefits Plans* covered trends in benefits and perquisites. Here are some trends we have noted in a broad span of industries, including healthcare.

- *Health insurance* is universal. Virtually all organizations use one or more type of plan, be it an indemnity, preferred provider organization (PPO), point of service (POS), or health maintenance organization (HMO) plan.
- *Life insurance* is provided by virtually all of the organizations. This may be based on a multiple of pay (79 percent) or a flat amount (11 percent).
- *Long-term disability* is provided by 96 percent of the respondents.
- *Accidental death and dismemberment* (AD&D) is provided by over 92 percent of the participating organizations. Voluntary AD&D is provided by 45 percent of the participants.
- *Dental insurance* is provided by over 80 percent of participants.
- *Prescription reimbursement* is provided by over 70 percent of organizations, typically with a co-pay provision.
- *Employee assistance programs* (EAPs), offering intervention and treatment for substance abuse, are provided by 56 percent of the participants.
- *Vision plans* are provided by slightly over half of the participants.

The following executive-level benefits are also offered, but their prevalence is unknown because they are difficult to track. From our experience at Andersen, however, these benefits are fairly common.

- *Deferred compensation.* As discussed in Chapter 5, many organizations enable their executives to accumulate wealth by providing deferred compensation. These programs are often structured as supplemental executive retirement programs (SERPs).
- *Split-dollar insurance.* One type of deferred compensation, also discussed in Chapter 5, is split-dollar insurance. The programs are popular because of the build-up in cash value and the opportunity for the healthcare organization to recover its premium payments, albeit well into the future.
- *Other benefits.* Some existing benefits can be enhanced at the executive level. For example, it is not unusual for an executive to be granted a waiver on eligibility for the maximum vacation benefit, or to at least replicate the vacation or time-off policy of his or her previous employer. Likewise, organizations may pay the cost of relocation, education, and other expenses associated with work for the organization.

To gain perspective on the compensation practices of healthcare organizations, we analyzed healthcare organizations located in the United States. We focused on the following positions:

- Chief executive officer
- Chief operating officer
- Chief financial officer
- Top human resources officer
- Vice president of patient care

We based our analysis on information gathered from the most recent IRS 990 Form statements filed for each healthcare organization. We aged the data to January 1, 2002, using a rate of a 5 percent compensation increase per year. This information is not being offered as a benchmarking tool, but rather to highlight the different ways an organization can group and use this kind of data.

DEFINITIONS

Before presenting the information, the following definitions are necessary.

- *Mean (or average)* was calculated by summing the data and dividing by the number of data points. Depending on the range of data points, the average may be significantly affected by high or low outlying data points.
- *Percentile* indicates the percentage of executives or companies that is equal to or below a specified percentage. For example, if at the 75th percentile compensation for the CEO is $350,000, then 75 percent of companies provide compensation of $350,000 or less.
- *Median* is the 50th percentile. Therefore, 50 percent of the healthcare organizations reported numbers higher than the median, and 50 percent of the healthcare organizations reported numbers lower than the median.
- *Compensation* for executives is the compensation reported in Part V of the IRS 990 Form report. This typically includes all compensation paid to the executive (i.e., all cash compensation components).
- *Number of incumbents* indicates the total number of healthcare organizations that reported compensation information for the applicable executive (matched by title).
- *All data* reported in this section is rounded to the nearest hundred.

IRS 990 FORM

The information reported below is based on IRS Form 990, which not-for-profits must file annually with the IRS to maintain their tax-exempt status. The form requires not-for-profit organizations to document their eligibility for tax-exempt status and to provide detailed financial and program information. Most of the information provided in the form is available to the public. Organizations now have the option of posting the returns online.

The IRS 990 Forms are reviewed by regulatory bodies that monitor not-for-profit organizations' compliance with various laws. Potential donors may also review the forms, if they want more financial and program information about the organization. The completed forms are available to anyone who makes a request.

Examples of the information required on the IRS 990 Form include:

- Revenue
- Expenses
- Changes in net assets
- Fund balances
- Service accomplishments
- Officers' compensation
- Directors' compensation
- Trustees' compensation
- Key employees' compensation

ALL HEALTHCARE ORGANIZATIONS COMPARISON

We conducted a detailed analysis of the cash compensation levels for five commonly reported positions in the IRS 990 Form of each healthcare organization. The tables in Exhibits 2.1A to 2.1E below represent the 25th, 50th, 75th percentile, as well as the average

Exhibit 2.1A

Total Cash Compensation

Chief Executive Officer
All Healthcare Organizations

Data Projected to January 1, 2002

Number of Incumbents	Ranking	IRS 990 Form Reported Compensation
22	75th percentile	$568.0
	Average	505.8
	Median (50th percentile)	453.5
	25th percentile	301.2

Exhibit 2.1B

Total Cash Compensation
Chief Operating Officer
All Healthcare Organizations
Data Projected to January 1, 2002

Number of Incumbents	Ranking	IRS 990 Form Reported Compensation
12	75th percentile	$392.4*
	Average	394.1*
	Median (50th percentile)	351.4
	25th percentile	220.5

* The overall average in this case is higher than the 75th percentile. The authors have confirmed this result, caused by unusual data distribution patterns.

Exhibit 2.1C

Total Cash Compensation
Chief Financial Officer
All Healthcare Organizations
Data Projected to January 1, 2002

Number of Incumbents	Ranking	IRS 990 Form Reported Compensation
21	75th percentile	$252.2
	Average	264.5
	Median (50th percentile)	238.9
	25th percentile	204.9

Exhibit 2.1D

Total Cash Compensation
Top Human Resources Officer
All Healthcare Organizations
Data Projected to January 1, 2002

Number of Incumbents	Ranking	IRS 990 Form Reported Compensation
8	75th percentile	$226.8
	Average	193.4
	Median (50th percentile)	170.6
	25th percentile	143.6

Exhibit 2.1E

Total Cash Compensation
Vice President of Patient Care
All Healthcare Organizations
Data Projected to January 1, 2002

Number of Incumbents	Ranking	IRS 990 Form Reported Compensation
10	75th percentile	$193.7
	Average	175.1
	Median (50th percentile)	155.7
	25th percentile	140.8

compensation for each position for all the healthcare organizations included in this analysis.

Our analysis, as expected, found that median compensation levels for the executives varied significantly by role. The actual compensation levels for the executives in our analysis varied greatly as well. For example, the actual CEO compensation levels in this analysis ranged from approximately $236,000 to $1,300,000 per year. The organizations in the higher end of this range are large, best-in-class organizations with very complicated strategic business plans.

Exhibit 2.2A illustrates the applicable positions as a percentage of the CEO's salary.

LOCATION COMPARISON

To illustrate the different ways data can be represented, we divided compensation information found in the IRS 990 Forms for the healthcare organizations into two groups, rural and urban.

Exhibits 2.3A to 2.3D below represent the 25th, 50th, 75th percentile and the average compensation for each position for all the

Exhibit 2.2A

Average Total Compensation Compared to the CEO

Position	75th Percentile	50th Percentile	Average	25th Percentile
CEO	100%	100%	100%	100%
COO	69%	78%	78%	73%
CFO	44%	53%	52%	68%
Top, HR	40%	38%	38%	48%
VP, Patient Services	34%	34%	35%	47%

healthcare organizations included in this analysis, by location. For illustrative purposes, we used the CEO and CFO positions.

We can clearly see a significant difference between CEO pay in rural and urban settings. The average urban healthcare organization CEO, based on this analysis, is paid over twice as much as a CEO in a rural setting, while the urban CEO position is paid approximately 22 percent higher than the all healthcare organizations CEO average.

Again, we can clearly see the significant difference between CFO pay in rural and urban settings. The average urban healthcare organization CFO, based on this analysis, is paid approximately 60 percent higher than the CFO in a rural setting. However, the urban CFO position is paid just 12 percent more than the average CFO in all healthcare organizations.

The exhibts above illustrate the same data in two distinct ways. Exhibit 2.3C includes all healthcare organizations and Exhibit 2.3D separates healthcare organizations by location. The results vary significantly.

Exhibits 2.4A and 2.4B show the compensation information for the CEO. Exhibit 2.4A shows the data with the single highest and

Exhibit 2.3A

Total Cash Compensation
Chief Executive Officer
Rural
Data Projected to January 1, 2002

Number of Incumbents	*Ranking*	*IRS 990 Form Reported Compensation*
8	75th percentile	$309.0
	Average	308.2
	Median (50th percentile)	302.8
	25th percentile	289.2

Exhibit 2.3B

Total Cash Compensation
Chief Executive Officer
Urban
Data Projected to January 1, 2002

Number of Incumbents	*Ranking*	*IRS 990 Form Reported Compensation*
14	75th percentile	$681.7
	Average	618.8
	Median (50th percentile)	526.7
	25th percentile	477.4

Exhibit 2.3C

Total Cash Compensation
Chief Financial Officer
Rural
Data Projected to January 1, 2002

Number of Incumbents	Ranking	IRS 990 Form Reported Compensation
7	75th percentile	$223.6
	Average	190.3
	Median (50th percentile)	184.5
	25th percentile	160.7

Exhibit 2.3D

Total Cash Compensation
Chief Financial Officer
Urban
Data Projected to January 1, 2002

Number of Incumbents	Ranking	IRS 990 Form Reported Compensation
14	75th percentile	$340.8
	Average	301.7
	Median (50th percentile)	240.6
	25th percentile	232.9

Exhibit 2.4A

Total Cash Compensation
Chief Executive Officer
Excluding Highest and Lowest Paid
Data Projected to January 1, 2002

Number of Incumbents	Ranking	IRS 990 Form Reported Compensation
20	75th percentile	$540.5
	Average	478.3
	Median (50th percentile)	453.5
	25th percentile	304.4

Exhibit 2.4B

Total Cash Compensation
Chief Executive Officer
Excluding Two Highest and Lowest Paid
Data Projected to January 1, 2002

Number of Incumbents	Ranking	IRS 990 Form Reported Compensation
20	75th percentile	$526.7
	Average	450.2
	Median (50th percentile)	453.5
	25th percentile	305.9

lowest paid incumbents excluded, while Exhibit 2.4B shows the data with the two highest and lowest paid incumbents excluded.

Interestingly, in Exhibits 2.4A and 2.4B, the 75th and 25th percentiles do not drop dramatically, but there is a significant change in the 75th percentile. Exhibits 2.5A and 2.5B show trends for CFOs.

In Exhibits 2.5A and 2.5B, the 75th percentile and 25th percentile drop a bit more than the CEO analysis; again they do not differ dramatically.

So far, we have outlined three different ways to use the same data:

1. All healthcare organizations
2. Locations (rural vs. urban)
3. Excluding outliers (exclude highest and lowest paid; exclude two highest and lowest paid)

Exhibit 2.6A shows the average CEO and CFO compensation information for each distinct way we represented the compensation data in our analysis as a percentage of the all healthcare organizations' data.

Exhibit 2.5A

Total Cash Compensation
Chief Financial Officer
Excluding Highest and Lowest Paid
Data Projected to January 1, 2002

Number of Incumbents	Ranking	IRS 990 Form Reported Compensation
19	75th percentile	$246.5
	Average	253.6
	Median (50th percentile)	238.9
	25th percentile	206.0

Exhibit 2.5B

Total Cash Compensation
Chief Financial Officer
Excluding Two Highest and Lowest Paid
Data Projected to January 1, 2002

Number of Incumbents	Ranking	IRS 990 Form Reported Compensation
17	75th percentile	$240.9
	Average	246.5
	Median (50th percentile)	238.9
	25th percentile	207.0

Exhibit 2.6A

Summary of Average Compensation
As a Percentage of All Healthcare Organizations

Position	All Organizations Healthcare	Location		Outliers	
		Rural	Urban	Excluding Highest Paid and Lowest Paid	Excluding 2 Highest Paid and 2 Lowest Paid
CEO	100%	61%	122%	92%	85%
CFO	100%	72%	114%	96%	93%

Not surprisingly, we found great variances in compensation within each position in this analysis. Many different factors can influence these differences in compensation levels, including the level of responsibility of the position, the size of the facility, and strategic business goals and objectives.

CHAPTER 3

Assessing Top Executive Leadership Performance: New Horizons

James A. Landry and Ralph D. Feigin

AS EVOLUTION PERSISTS both in the business world and in medical science, the top executive leaders of healthcare institutions face a clear leadership challenge. In every sector of healthcare—from local hospitals, medical schools, and academic health science centers to the most far-flung healthcare multinationals—new market and scientific forces are increasing the pressure to deliver more meaningful, results-oriented performance. How can they meet this challenge?

SIGNS OF THE TIMES

Meeting this challenge is not easy. In this time of profound business change, senior executives literally shoulder the burden of the future. As stewards, they must chart the course for their organizations, successfully articulating vision and mission while implementing vital strategic objectives—including customer service, process improvement, human capital management, research and development—and ensuring returns on all these areas of investment. They must demonstrate sharply honed and exceptional skills by optimizing available resources to beat the competition. In so doing, they must strengthen their organizations' financial viability with minimal risk.

But top executive leadership performance is not just about getting the "right business results." Successful performance is also tied directly to creating, nurturing, and maintaining the "right culture," that is, the right ways of thinking, working, and doing. It is about building and sustaining "the place" where the best results happen—a place where people are prepared to meet current challenges and contribute innovative solutions for present and future opportunities. To focus only on results "suffocates the spirit," as Russ S. Moxley (2000) notes in his recent book on *Leadership and Spirit*.

Healthcare is not immune from the challenges of the day, from which trends emerge and business risks arise. In *The Cultural Creatives,* Paul H. Ray and Sherry Ruth Anderson (2000) claim that visionaries and futurists are predicting a long-anticipated change in the way we do business and politics. They call it a "demand for authenticity," which means a change in worldview, life priorities, and lifestyle, such as how we spend our time and money. If we look at workforce trends (see Figure 3.1) we can easily recognize the manifestations of such change, e.g., loyalty to career versus to the organization, the valuing of a balanced work-life, and a sense of urgency to succeed. We are in the "midst of epochal change," according to Ray and Anderson, "caught between globalization, accelerating technologies, and deteriorating planetary ecology." Peter Senge's (2001) position on the "future state" is stated as, "perhaps no time in history has afforded greater possibilities for a collective change in direction" (Senge and Goran 2001).

As we approach the horizon of this truly "new economy" we realize the rules of the game have, indeed, changed. The new economy is not merely the economy of the Internet we have known for the past decade. Rather, it is the profoundly new business world that the Internet and other technologies have made possible.

The hallmarks of the day are speed, flexibility, and innovation—at a reasonable value-added cost and the highest quality. Business

Figure 3.1: Workforce Trends

Out: loyal employees and employers
In: war for talent (putting contracts through the "shredder")

Out: rigid pay scales
In: flexible compensation and work arrangements

Out: reward for seniority and effort
In: reward for competencies and results

Out: power structure
In: inclusion

Out: locker room climates
In: gender-balanced workforce (women nearly fully absorbed)

Out: 9 to 5 in one time zone
In: 24/7 in all time zones (inter-econ work whenever customers are awake)

Out: old guard mentoring
In: workers negotiating and networking their own way through careers

Out: internal equity
In: person-based pay

Out: holding onto jobs forever in fear of losing "two comma income"
In: retiring at 40

Out: labor shortage
In: new pools of employees (e.g., high-talent disabled, immigrant, offshore)

and, thus, healthcare executive leadership, must be "flexible, nimble, and responsive with a host of forces working against them," say Michael E. Raynor and Joseph L. Bower (2001) in a recent *Harvard Business Review* article. Global interconnectedness will intensify as business cycles widen to become worldwide in scale. New institutional structures in finance and investment will emerge, thereby changing norms and policies. Organizational structures will become more organic—resembling molecular lattices rather than boxes or pyramids.

One telltale sign of this new economy is occupational change. It is estimated that almost a third of all new jobs are now in flux (i.e., dying, being born, added, or subtracted). In *Rewarding Excellence,* Edward E. Lawler and Susan A. Mohrman (1998) state that "virtually every product and service is in surplus"—shifting power from sellers to buyers and transferring power from employer to employee.

HEALTHCARE TRENDS

In healthcare, external factors have had a powerful effect on internal cultures. Healthcare continues to undergo a massive transformation as an industry due to such factors as technological advancements, managed care, and outpatient treatments. In his article "Pay for Performance," Gordon Hawthorne (2000) cites Moody's *1999 Outlook and Medians for Not-For-Profit Healthcare,* which predicts a bumpy road for healthcare in the near term because of increased revenue pressure, merger and acquisition integration risk factors, and efforts to terminate or restructure strategies that are proving costly.

Over the next three to five years volatility and risks may increase as healthcare organizations assimilate newly acquired cultures, change physician relationships, expand into new business lines, and reach out to new—including foreign—sources of capital. Lowell Johnson, CFO, Providence Health System, in an interview with *Healthcare Financial Management* claims that for the next 10 years, "the single largest challenge facing healthcare" is the "lack of a national health policy in America" (Johnson 2000). He claims that this lack of policy has placed an undue burden on Medicaid and Medicare, even while the financial resources of both individuals and organizations shrink (growing at a rate lower than the rate of inflation). The challenge will be to provide quality care with these limited resources in the face of escalating costs.

These enormous changes and challenges raise the bar for healthcare's top executive leadership performance. Some of the critical challenges facing healthcare leadership include:

- Meeting increasing demands with strained resources.
- Bridging academic, research, clinical, and administrative cultures.
- Effectively integrating new technology.
- Learning and applying best practices of other healthcare and nonhealthcare institutions.
- Developing expanded leadership capability.
- Responding proactively to pressures for quality, cost-effective, efficient services.
- Applying excellent solutions leveraging "breakthrough knowledge" for healthcare delivery.

Every organization, including every healthcare organization, wants to have in place—or be positioned to develop—innovative and visionary leadership to drive their business forward, maintaining or gaining competitive ground. Top executive leaders are the "single most powerful faction behind change," notes Jac Fitz-enz (1997) in his book on exceptional companies. Executive leadership must achieve—and even better exceed—an ever-expanding business vision, continually recalibrating and reenergizing performance in the quest for best results. As Hawthorne (2000) warns, "Boards have become less tolerant of delivering margins, faded efforts to achieve consolidation efficiencies, and losses." It all adds up to this: Top executive leadership today must be able do the right thing right at the right time each and every time.

Our focus in this writing is on the role of the leader and the leadership team—those responsible to ensure that the organization meets the challenge of change through attention and commitment to values, culture, vision, mission, and goals.

There is a clear distinction between the role of leadership and that of management. In his highly regarded book *On Becoming A Leader,* Warren Bennis (1989) distinguishes between these two roles (see Figure 3.2). For Bennis, this distinction is not necessarily an "either/or; one can be both a good manager and fine leader. Not all good managers, however, are good leaders and vice versa. The tasks and roles are strikingly different, as are the competencies, performance, and functional/process accountability." The following discussion should make this clear.

LEADERS AS COMPASSIONATE AGENTS OF CHANGE

Performance success implies change, which, in turn, requires the ability to tolerate uncertainty, ambiguity, and unpredictability. If an organization continues to conduct "business as usual," the company will suffer. At best it will be mediocre; at worst it will fail. Top performing leaders, of course—inherently and from pressures of both internal and external forces—are never satisfied with the status quo or being just competitive. They are compelled to "lead the pack"—be "best in show" and viewed as "world class." To achieve such prominent ranking requires executive leadership first and foremost to serve as the leading agent of change, determining what changes must be made and shaping the initiatives needed to continuously optimize organizational performance. It also means assessing and managing the human impact of change.

How change is managed—that is, planned, created, and led—determines what changes will ultimately occur and potentially succeed. The ability to manage change is the single most critical competency required of leaders today. Certainly healthcare leaders must possess this ability, as they and their people strive to increase patient satisfaction, decrease the cycle time for case work, introduce new medical technology, and make the tough decisions—including cutting operating expenses in mid-stream of a project.

Figure 3.2: Manager vs. Leader

- The manager administers; the leader innovates.
- The manager is a copy; the leader is an original.
- The manager focuses on systems and structure; the leader focuses on people.
- The manager relies on control; the leader inspires trust.
- The manager has a short-range view; the leader has a long-range perspective.
- The manager asks how and when; the leader asks what and why.
- The manager has his eye always on the bottom line; the leader has his eye on the horizon.
- The manager imitates; the leader originates.
- The manager accepts the status quo; the leader challenges it.
- The manager is the classic good soldier; the leader is his own person.
- The manager does things right; the leader does the right thing.

Source: Bennis, W. 1989. *On Becoming a Leader.* Reading, MA: Addison-Wesley.

As these leaders change a current business process or organization reporting relationship, they must prepare to explain "why." Whenever change is introduced, it sparks resistance, because it threatens existing modes of behavior, attitudes, and relationships. Leaders must understand barriers to change and know how to overcome resistance in positive ways. They must know how to help people implement predetermined changes and move through the psychological impact of change, thus making behavior change a driver and not an outcome

LEADING BY EXAMPLE

The top executive leadership team (not just selected executives) must be the first to demonstrate, through collective behavior and continuous performance improvement, that there is a new way of doing business. Such elements as strategy, culture, competencies, and performance must be aligned to executive team compensation and behavior to maximize results.

Recognizing that strong leadership is essential for survival in today's competitive environment, Valerie Sessa and Jodi Taylor (2000), in their book *Executive Selection*, draw on years of research and over 1,000 interviews by the Center for Creative Leadership pertaining to executive selection. They concur that choosing the "right" top level executives is the most important strategic decision that can be made by the organization. Sessa and Taylor proclaim "it is not the consequence or results of the action but the action itself" that is "wholly under the control" of the top executives. Michael Treacy and Fred Wiersema (1995) underscore the importance of executive selection. It is a way of building the future, "not a marketing plan, public relations campaign, or a way to chat up stockholders."

Burt Nanus (1989) in *The Leaders Edge: The Seven Keys to Leadership in a Turbulent World* develops in great detail the general characteristics required to fill a top leadership role: "Leaders take charge, make things happen, dream dreams, and then translate them into reality. Leaders attract the voluntary commitment of followers, energize them, and transform organizations into new entities with greater potential for survival, growth and excellence. Effective leadership empowers an organization to maximize its contribution to the well being of its members and the larger society of which it is a part. If managers are known for their skills in solving problems, then leaders are known for being masters in designing and building institutions; they are the architects of the organization's future."

VALUES, CULTURE, VISION, MISSION, AND GOALS

The fusion of values, culture, vision, and mission provide the overarching context for future goals, defining the purpose of a change initiative and organization direction flow.

Top healthcare executive leadership faces challenges, dilemmas, and, ultimately, choices every day. They must create the templates for strategic direction and organization performance. Executive leadership must continue to prune business activities that no longer fit the "value-creation logic" of strategic goals. They must also integrate new strategic goals, to quote Robert Burgelman and Yves L. Doz (2001), by "combining resources and competencies from business units and directing them towards ... exploiting existing and new opportunities simultaneously."

Leaders must also accept accountability for individual and team success in creating the desired future. As Edgar H. Schein has observed in many of his writings, leaders wield significant influence over employees, simply by where they ask them to focus their attention. Leaders, says Schein, are "the undisputed critical players in improving an organization's performance—especially if significant improvement is the goal."

As leaders lead new initiatives, they must know how to inspire action. A new vision cannot catch on or take hold if clashes with the organization's basic assumptions, paradigms, and values. Indeed, such a mismatch is one of the most frequent causes of resistance to change.

Organizational values play a key role here. They provide the context within which leaders and their people identify key issues and evaluate or change goals. Values shape assumptions about the future and limit the range of choices considered for a new vision. Values determine whether a new sense of direction will be enthusiastically embraced, reluctantly accepted, or rejected out of hand.

An organization's culture also plays an important part in the paradigm of change. Culture generates and assimilates an organization's values and as such constitutes an organizational memory that guides behavior. It is both map and compass, providing a sense of identity, stability, and boundaries.

The vision of an organization is a comprehensive picture (oftentimes literally) of the desired future state of the organization. Vision is decidedly one particular "future" out of many possible choices.

It captures the essence of the core values and characteristics (e.g., processes, structure, systems, people, and skills) of the "ideal place" described in the beginning of this chapter.

The vision is also the precursor to the stated mission. Moxley (2000), in his book on leadership, notes that a leader must articulate the organization's vision "compellingly, in a way that truly engages followers." It is the organization vision that creates the strongest sense of connectedness for all employees. "Where there is no vision, the people perish." (Proverbs 29:18).

In articulating the mission of an organization, leaders should strive to convey to all stakeholders the basic purpose or reason for the organization's existence—what the organization is striving "to be." The mission is an aspirational statement that in very general terms describes what the organization does; but more importantly, focuses on its value to society. A mission describes the unique position an organization aspires to achieve in its field, and what it takes for the organization to succeed (see Figure 3.3).

COMPETENCY: A KEY INGREDIENT IN PERFORMANCE SUCCESS

Top executive leadership is grounded in competence. The most typical definition of "competence" is the effective application of knowledge, skills, and abilities by an individual. This definition is often expanded to include organizational, team, and/or functional areas. Defined in these ways, competence must also include behavioral characteristics at the individual, team, and/or organization level. In the right combination and for the right set of circumstances, such characteristics predict superior performance and/or attributes. L. M. Spencer and S. M. Spencer (1993) define competency as an "underlying characteristic of an individual that is causally related to criterion-referenced effective and/or superior performance in a job or situation." They continue their expansion

Figure 3.3: Example Mission Statements

Bard (C.R. Bard, Inc.)
Leading multinational developer, manufacturer,
and marketer of health care products.

STATEMENT | Mission

Bard's Mission is to advance the delivery of health care by profitably developing, manufacturing, and marketing value-driven products which meet the quality, integrity, and service expectations of our customers while providing opportunities for employees. As a result, we will optimize shareholder value and be a respected worldwide health care company.

Southwest Airlines Co.
Single-class airline primarily serving shorthaul city pairs.

STATEMENT | Mission

The mission of Southwest Airlines is dedication to the highest quality of Customer Service delivered with a sense of warmth, friendliness, individual pride, and company Spirit.

To Our Employees

We are committed to provide our employees a stable work environment with equal opportunity for learning and personal growth. Creativity and innovation are encouraged for improving the effectiveness of Southwest Airlines. Above all, employees will be provided the same concern, respect, and caring attitude within the organization that they are expected to share externally with every Southwest Customer.

Pfizer
Research-based pharmaceutical company with global operations.

STATEMENT | Mission

Over the next five years, we will achieve and sustain our place as the world's premier research-based health care company. Our continuing success as a business will benefit patients and our customers, our shareholders, our families, and the communities in which we operate around the world.

In each of its global health care businesses, Pfizer will secure a leading position through excellence in the following areas:

- Research and development.
- Marketing innovative products.
- Finanacial performance.

Continental Medical Systems, Inc.
Diversified provider of comprehensive medical
rehabilitation and physician services.

STATEMENT | Mission
Acting as a diversified provider of medical rehabilitation and physician activities, the Mission of Continental Medical Systems is to ensure high quality and cost effective outcomes to those we serve while providing a favorable return to our stockholders.

Source: Abrahams, J. 1999. *The Mission Statement Book: 301 Corporate Mission Statements from America's Top Companies.* Berkeley, CA: Ten Speed Press.

by defining competencies as having five key characteristics, which are a fairly deep and an enduring part of a person's personality:

1. *Motives:* The things a person consistently thinks about or wants, and that cause action. *Example:* Achievement-motivated people consistently set challenging goals for themselves, taking personal responsibility for accomplishing them and using feedback to do better.
2. *Physical traits:* Physical characteristics and consistent responses to situations or information. *Example:* Reaction time and good eyesight are physical trait competencies of combat pilots.
3. *Self-Concept:* A person's attitudes, values, or images in relation to the person's own self. *Example:* Self-confidence, a person's belief that he or she can be effective in almost any situation, is part of that person's concept of self.

4. *Knowledge:* Information a person has in specific content areas. *Example:* A surgeon's knowledge of nerves and muscles in the human body constitutes a knowledge-based competency.
5. *Skill:* The ability to perform a certain physical or mental task. *Example:* A computer programmer's key skill is the ability to efficiently organize lines of code in logical sequential order.

Significantly, Spencer and Spencer (1993) include behavior in their definition of competence, not limiting competence to knowledge, skills, and abilities. Clearly, these latter elements are important but typically only the "tip of the iceberg." They are easily observed and measured, but there is significantly more to competence than only what you see "above the water line." These are the "surface elements of competence" as David McClellan (1976) points out in his classic guide to job assessment. McClellan also states, however, it is what is below the surface, that is, "the belief systems and motives," that are the core competencies. Core competencies are the "vital few" competencies—the combined set of skills, knowledge, abilities, and behavioral characteristics—that will bring about optimal performance and results.

Thomas Teal's *Harvard Business Review* article (1996) "The Human Side of Management" begins by noting a paradox about leadership. It looks easy—so easy that we all think we can succeed where others fail. Yet Teal points out that true leadership requires a profound contribution to an organization. Executive leadership is expected to demonstrate performance success in finance, product development, marketing, technology, strategy, negotiation and so forth. In addition, it involves much more than technique. "It magnifies the social core of human nature, brings individual talents to fruition, creates value—injects passion to generate advantages for every member of the organization's team" (Teal 1996).

Executive leadership, in Teal's view, means swimming against the current—against the wish of one or more constituents. It means facing and at times defying convention, criticism, and even heavy odds. Though Teal does not use the term "core competence," he does use words such as persuasion, ingenuity, tenacity, courage, integrity, imagination, wit, loyalty, personal responsibility, compassion, humanitarian, vision, compunction, morals, and mentoring—all of which could easily describe leadership competencies

LEADERSHIP COMPETENCY: SHARPENING THE SAW

Stephen Covey's remarkable book about the human condition, *The 7 Habits of Highly Effective People* (1989), presents the brief story of one man encountering another in the woods working feverishly to saw down a tree. Noticing that the logger is exhausted after many hours of sawing without much success, the man asks him why he does not stop to sharpen the saw. "I don't have time to sharpen the saw," the man says emphatically. "I'm too busy sawing."

This story relates to Covey's Habit 7, the habit of "renewal." Covey suggests that through continuous improvement, people can attain new levels of understanding and consequently move to a "higher plane." The moral is clear: If you "sharpen the saw," you can achieve such heights sooner rather than later. As leaders set an organization's vision, articulate its mission, and identify and align key strategic goals, they in effect define what the organization will do. The focus now shifts to *how* the performance will be achieved. Leadership competencies are the tools that sharpen the saw to achieve higher level results and fulfill the vision and mission.

To perform we must have something to perform against. To evaluate performance, organizations need to employ a "mixed model" of performance. Such a model combines both the goal and the path—both the results leaders are expected to achieve and the competencies that they must posses to achieve them. One good guide to such competencies is Fitz-enz's *8 Practices of Highly Spiritual Companies* (1997). In this book, Fitz-enz outlines determinants of exceptional executive leadership performance based on an analysis of approximately 1,000 successful companies, including healthcare organizations. His findings indicate that organizations featuring the following characteristics consistently outperform the "competition" (Fitz-enz 1997):

- *Value:* constant effort to add value and not simply do something.
- *Commitment:* dedication to long-term success, not the latest fad.
- *Culture:* always looking for ways to link organizational values to operational systems.
- *Commitment:* extraordinary concern for communication with all stakeholders.
- *Partnering with stakeholders:* new ways of doing business to meet new market conditions and customer requirements.
- *Collaboration:* collective support and cohesiveness across sections.
- *Innovation and risk:* willingness to shake up the organization and start anew or rebuild.
- *Competitive passion:* constantly searching for improvement and selling ideas.

The work of Fitz-enz regarding organization competencies is an exceptionally good template from which to build and bridge specific core competencies for top executive leadership in healthcare. Competency research studies conducted by human capital and organization development consultants have identified core competencies most important to top executive leadership across industries. Each competency requires a well-defined set of behaviors and, thereby, establishes clear criteria for leadership selection and performance recognition and development (see Figure 3.4).

Leadership competencies express the expected and required behaviors of the organization as seen through the vision, heard through the mission, and operationalized through the strategic goals and tactics.

In *Leadership Without Easy Answers,* Ronald Heifetz (1994) outlines several categories of internal and external responsibilities that should be assessed for top executives. They include both quantitative (business) and qualitative (behavioral) results—the "what," such

Figure 3.4: Leadership Core Competencies

- Facilitating others
- Self confidence and direction
- Trusted influence
- Interpersonal understanding
- Initiative and risk taking
- Business acumen
- Customer value orientation
- Organizational awareness
- Compelling vision

- Relationship building
- Continuous quality improvement
- Teamwork and collaboration
- Achievement orientation
- Direct persuasion
- Developing others
- Conceptual/innovative thinking
- Change enablement
- **Focused business drive**

Competency Example: Focused Business Drive

Definition: The demonstrated ability to create, generate, and capitalize on business development ideas and opportunities for competitive advantage.

Behaviors
- Displays a high concern and regard for setting standards of excellence.
- Stays focused on relevant business market information and conditions with a keen focus on future business opportunities.
- Strives to develop and achieve sound and ambitious business development goals.
- Continually looks for new and viable ways of doing business to add value for the customer.
- Commits necessary resources to act decisively to make things happen.

as financial performance, market share, quality, daily operations, charitable care rendered, health promotion, and education delivered; and the "how," such as management style and relations with medical staff, board members, employees, and community leaders.

Based on the work of Heifetz as well as extensive survey research, the American College of Healthcare Executives (ACHE), along with the American Hospital Association, and the American Medical Association, and Ernst & Young, concluded that the most important competency of a successful leader is the ability to resolve conflict. In their 1996 *Study of the Roles and Working Relationships of the Hospital Board Chairman, CEO, and Medical Staff President; Executive Summary,* they asserted that the successful healthcare leader:

- "Identifies the adaptive challenge" (i.e., immediately recognizes issues in a situation and determines how to solve them).
- "Regulates stress" (i.e., knows the level of distress in his/her organization and acts to relieve it).
- "Directs disciplined attention to issues" (i.e., thinks through all aspects of a problem and makes appropriate decisions).
- "Gives the work to the stakeholders" (i.e., recognizes that every problem within the organization has its own stakeholders who should be involved in seeking solutions).
- "Protects the voices of community leadership" (i.e., ensures that all those in the community with a stake in an issue are heard).

In an earlier report, ACHE (1993) established three important categories for top executive leadership ability and performance accountability, as illustrated in Figure 3.5.

Figure 3.6 shows how these categories may be expressed as competencies for the purposes of leadership evaluation.

PERFORMANCE ASSESSMENT: STEPS TO SUCCESS

So how does all this add up to a performance assessment system? Performance assessment—managing and leading people by providing feedback and direction related to actions expected and taken—can be the single greatest challenge for the hospital or medical school board and/or members of the executive leadership team. In a recent article in *Journal of Healthcare Management,* John F. Newman and coauthors (2001) shed light on why it can be so difficult. Their research shows that the difficulty of appraisal (and

Figure 3.5: ACHE Major Areas of Evaluation

Area-wide Health Status
- Community healthcare improvement
- Healthcare management
- Trends/assessment
- Social service projects/policy

Institutional Success
- Planning (charting future; drive long-/short-term plan)
- Human resource management (optimizing human capital)
- Quality of services (total quality management, or TQM, advocate)
- Fiscal management (resource allocation that is cost effective and fiscally responsible)
- Compliance with regulations (licensing, accreditation, quality assurance)
- Advocacy (influencing legislative/regulatory policy)
- Organizational promotion (community integration, public relations, business leader involvement)
- Leadership ability (clear vision, ability to communicate)

Professional Role Fulfillment
- Professional currency (staying abreast of professional developments)
- Professional advancement
- Continuing education
- Professional involvement
- Ethics

hence the quality of most appraisals) grows proportionally with the increase in the level of executive responsibility.

But in spite of the challenges, assessment must occur; it is both inevitable and important. Today, as in the past, leaders must be held accountable for their leadership. This process of accountability can bring significant benefits to an organization; the value of performance management:

Figure 3.6: Competency Examples

Planning
Definition: The demonstrated ability to plan, direct, and monitor activities that continuously and noticeably improve the organization's products, programs, processes, and services.

Behaviors
- Monitors key internal and external trends, opportunities, and "at risk" potentials.
- Accurately assesses the strength, weaknesses, opportunities, and threats ("SWOT") to ensure proper course of action for organizational advancement.
- Evaluates the organizational resources and capabilities to address and implement change.
- Provides astute and workable approaches and methodologies to achieve desired results in an accurate and timely manner.
- Anticipates proactively any problems with the organization's process, structure, and resource allocation, and provides effective "best practice" tactics for corrective action.

Customer Value Orientation
Definition: The demonstrated ability to maintain a constant and consistent focus on all customer needs in order to provide the highest value of service with an exceptional level of satisfaction.

Behaviors
- Maintains a sharp focus on needs and requirements of internal and external customers.
- Closely tracks customer expectations and requirements and makes timely, effective, and efficient interventions based on changing needs.
- Continuously clarifies, improves, and applies new ways to add value for the customer.

- Demonstrates the board is overseeing top leadership performance.
- Links strategic goals to the business plan.
- Aligns leadership and stakeholder interests.

- Establishes accountability to stakeholders.
- Aligns the business culture with performance requirements.
- Sets targets for optimal levels of achievement.
- Improves retention and productivity.
- Detects early signs of performance problems.
- Creates a sense of teamwork.
- Inspires and accelerates improved performance through feedback and counsel.
- Creates empowerment, shared responsibility, and "ownership."
- Communicates the "whats" and "hows" of role and work.
- Sets clear expectations and key performance indicators for success.
- Stimulates innovation.
- Provides a sound basis for meaningful rewards.
- Ensures compliance to any regulatory requirements.
- Reinforces common identity and culture.

Newman et al. (2001) put forth the premise that healthcare organizations must conduct leadership assessment to:

1. determine if the individual is performing to expectations;
2. account for how well and how conscientiously the leadership team members are performing;
3. defend from legal actions;
4. facilitate board–CEO communication regarding expectation;
5. assess improvement opportunities and "detect warning signs; and
6. create a sense of teamwork.

Performance assessment is a way to change behavior, increase understanding, communicate the need for change, manage expectations, link to reward and recognition, substantiate the right focus, create a sense of ownership, define success, and guide organizational, team, and individual direction and achievement goals.

A key to an effective top executive leadership resides in a dynamic process which includes five critical steps:

1. setting key performance indicators;
2. planning and executing;
3. monitoring and evaluating;
4. rewarding and recognizing; and
5. coaching and developing.

Step 1: Set key performance indicators

So far we have discussed the leader as a leading agent of change and as the keeper of the faith in values, culture, vision, mission, and goals. As leaders strive to direct these elements harmoniously, they need to set key *performance indicators,* for success must be driven from the top executive leadership throughout the organization. Key performance indicators are the measurable and observable results of behavior, that is, competencies (see Figure 3.7). The primary strategic goals that an organization chooses will define the right type and balance of such competencies. Leaders must establish these goals as performance measures, and cascade them throughout the organization. In this way, they effectively operationalize the future state pictured in the vision and pledged in the mission.

Top executive leaders must know in advance how their performance will be defined and measured, setting clear threshold levels for expected results. They are also the measurements of time, quality, cost, and quantity (i.e., output and process measures).

Output and/or process of key performance indicators for top executive leadership are most typically aligned to organizational and team metrics such as profit, return on equity, growth, results versus budget/operating plan, customer opinion, and customer relation. These indicators are the results or "what," but not the "how"(i.e., the competencies which drive and influence these results).

Figure 3.7: Key Performance Indicator (KPI) Characteristics

• Linked to objectives	Can the measure be aligned with an objective?
• Controllable/influenceable	Can the results be controlled or significantly influenced under a span of responsibility?
• Actionable	Can action be taken to improve performance?
• Simple	Can the measure be easily and clearly explained?
• Credible	Is the measure resistant to manipulation?
• Integrated	Can the measure be linked both down and across the organization?
• Measurable	Can the measure be quantified?

Several new theories have emerged and corresponding models developed regarding the balance of key output metrics. The most widely regarded and implemented is the Balanced Scorecard™ developed by Robert Kaplan and Donald Norton (1996).

Like similar approaches, the Balanced Scorecard moves beyond the limited financial emphasis of the past. It supplements financial measures because such measures look backward, not forward; they are lag—not lead—indicators. Because they focus on historical inputs rather than future outputs, financial numbers, taken alone, lack predictive power. Although they are the most important of all indicators, they need to be seen in a more balanced perspective that includes nonfinancial key performance indicators.

The Kaplan-Norton scorecard includes four perspectives, covering financial performance, customer relations, internal processes, and, learning and growth. Most organizations that have adopted a Balanced Scorecard approach to executive leadership performance assessment "populate" these four perspectives with their highest-priority performance indicators.

Some organizations have adapted the scorecard to best fit their needs and requirements. For example, Duke Children's Hospital developed a Research, Education, and Teaching perspective instead of "learning and growth." Montefiore Hospital's Balanced Scorecard established an adaptation to reflect a "new strategy launch" to become more efficient and customer-focused, and to increase market share with new products and services.

Kaplan and Norton (2001) point out that when assessing senior management performance, healthcare institutions, in comparison to other kinds of companies, tend to pay more attention to customers. In his survey of healthcare CEOs and medical school department chairs, J. L. Tyler (1994) found that these leaders used a variety of assessment tools. Although nearly 90 percent of the leaders ranked financial results as the most important performance measure, they did not stop there. Communication was second, followed by integrity, resource management, compliance, quality initiatives, accreditation results, community health, and customer satisfaction.

The Value Dynamics model depicted in Figure 3.8 also includes nonfinancial measures in multiple perspectives. This model features five perspectives: physical, financial, customer, employee/supplier, and organization. Measures here include quality of strategy (from concept to execution), credibility of leadership, talent of workforce, innovation, and market share.

Whichever model healthcare leaders use, it is important to use a performance assessment model that includes nonfinancial measures. Only then can leaders operationalize their institution's vision and mission.

Step 2: Plan and Execute

The key performance indicators tell only half the story in terms of performance expectations and assessment by focusing on results. The other half is how to do it—that is, how to encourage the

Figure 3.8: Value Dynamics Framework

Financial	Physical	Customer	Employee & Suppliers	Organization
Strategic financial management	Efficient systems	Patient centered	Employer of choice	Brand recognition
Strategic financial position Manage unit costs.	Grow capacity to meet demand	Provide quality physicians	Improve physician retention	Build CHS brand recognition
Improve A/R processes	Address patient wait time	Conduct satisfaction survey	Identify dissatisfaction areas	Conduct brand survey
Implement benchmarking	Assess capacity	Monitor recruitment initiatives	Monitor retention initiatives	Define the market
% net revenue collected	Clinical cost per unit	Average length of stay	Physician employee satisfaction	Market share growth
Accounts receivable cycle time	Inventory turns	Patient Satisfaction	Physician retention	% growth in new patients

required competencies. Planning and executing performance requires dialogue. Leaders and those who oversee them must agree on the competencies (not just results) that will be used as performance indicators. Such competencies might include particular kinds of knowledge, skills, abilities, and behavioral attributes.

Typically, the board would define the core competencies required for the CEO, and the CEO would, in turn, define the core competencies for the medical staff president (in hospitals), and, as applicable, the other top executive leadership team members or "C" level offices (e.g., chief operating officer, chief financial officer, chief human resources officer, and chief information officer).

After identifying expected competencies as well as target results, top executive leaders must "attach themselves" to these expectations. There must be a plan of action to effectively execute the performance expectations. While executive leadership must know what and how to delegate to let others grow and mature, they must also accept full responsibility for their own success.

Step 3: Monitor and Evaluate

An affective assessment program requires continuous monitoring to ensure that all in the organization are striving to achieve the right results in the right way. Actions should support organizational strategy. All managers (including senior managers) should work to increase the value of their human capital. This means giving, receiving, and documenting ongoing feedback, providing development opportunities, and appraising performance on schedule. The entire system should be working to improve individual, team, and organization performance. The following checklist offers guidelines for monitoring effectiveness.

- The system is understood and supported by top leadership and the board, who consider it effective.
- The system includes a detailed administration manual.
- The system is supported by an official policy on performance assessment.
- The system is simple and easy to administer.
- The system requires managers to complete and give performance assessments on schedule.

- The system is used as a tool to improve individual, team, and organizational performance.

In addition, top leadership must continuously strive to control the pace of work, ensure efficient procedures, and hold people's "feet to the fire" to ensure results.

One effective and direct method to assess performance of top executive leadership is to develop and use assessment forms. Forms are not a substitute for the performance assessment process, but rather an adjunct and enhancement. The forms should include both results or outputs and competencies. Figure 3.9 offers a core competency assessment form. Typically, top leadership executives will have the same shared core competencies with additional key competencies unique to a particular role (i.e., CFO vs. COO). Similarly, executive leadership performance indicators should be delineated for each role; and, as with competencies, there may be certain indicators that are core or shared by more than one role. Both competencies and indicators, for example, can be put in a balanced scorecard format to stress strategic perspectives (e.g., financial, customer, process, research) and simply but effectively communicate strategic goals.

Step 4: Reward and Recognize

Reward and recognition enable top executives to "share in the success" of value-added results. According to Thomas L. Gilbert (1996) in *Human Competence,* those receiving such recognition are the "competent people" who create valuable results without using excessively costly behavior. What they give grows faster than what they receive.

Creating valuable results hinges on three key points (Gilbert 1996):

1. First, top executive leadership must believe the anticipated satisfaction of attaining higher-level results is greater than the current satisfaction with present results.

Figure 3.9: Core Competency Assessment Template

Competency	Unsatisfactory	Deficient	Fully Competent	Commendable	Exemplary
• Focused Business Drive					
Demonstrates the ability to create, generate, and capitalize on business development ideas and opportunities for competitive advantage.	○	○	○	○	○
Displays a high concern and regard for setting standards of excellence.	○	○	○	○	○
Stays focused on relevant business market information and conditions with a keen focus on future business opportunities.	○	○	○	○	○
Strives to develop and achieve sound and ambitious business development goals.	○	○	○	○	○
Continually looks for new and viable ways of doing business to add value for the customer. Commits necessary resources to act decisively to make things happen.	○	○	○	○	○

continued

Figure 3.9: *(continued)*

- Planning

Demonstrates the ability to plan, direct, and monitor activities and to continuously and noticeably improve the organization's products, programs, processes, and services.	○	○	○
Monitors key internal and external trends, opportunities, and "at risk" potentials.	○	○	○
Accurately assesses the strength, weaknesses, opportunities and threats to ensure proper course of action for organizational advancement.	○	○	○
Evaluates the organizational resources and capabilities to address and implement change.	○	○	○
Provides astute and workable approaches and methodologies to achieve desired results in an accurate and timely manner.	○	○	○
Anticipates proactively any problems with the organization's process, structure, and resource allocation and provide effective "best practice" tactics for corrective action.	○	○	○

- Additional core competencies as defined, for example:

Customer value orientation	○	○	○
Comfort resolution	○	○	○
Relationship building	○	○	○
Professional development	○	○	○

2. Second, top executive leadership must have a "can do attitude" about performing the results and consequences, believ-
   ing that reward and recognition are worth the effort (i.e., the
   "expectancy theory; see Figure 3.10).
3. Finally, there needs to be a "line of influence." In order to be
   motivated, as Lawler (2000) has observed, top executive
   leadership must see how their behavior influences a result
   that in turn deserves a reward.

Motivation is quite simply a source of energy. Like the elec-
trical currents in a battery, it has key elements such as amplitude
(how much), duration (how long), and velocity (how fast).
Motivational energy must be connected with or directed toward
a goal. The more attractive the goal (anticipated reward and recognition), the greater the energy (amplitude, duration, and velocity). Energy comes from two sources of value or valuing: intrinsic
and extrinsic. These two valuing sources serve as the basis for
reward and recognition.

Intrinsic valuing means that people inherently want to do a
good job and be recognized for it. It is in their nature to look for
challenges and the opportunity to grow and develop. In most
instances, the job satisfiers are not related to pay. People want to
enjoy what they do. They want a stimulating work environment
and the necessary resources to do their job and do it well. Effective
reward and recognition is based in fair and equitable pay, supple-
mented with noncash rewards. These include not only obvious
types of recognition such as promotion, but also positive and
timely feedback on a "job well done," public recognition, time
off, and certificates of achievement. In a university setting (such
as a teaching hospital), they may include the change to achieve
recognition through scholarly publication (in the university's medical journal), state-of-the-art research space, and, most valuable of
all, academic tenure.

Not all job satisfiers are, of course, intrinsic; many are extrinsic. The most common extrinsic source of satisfaction is money—

Figure 3.10: Expectancy Theory

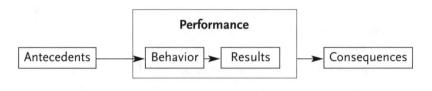

especially money earned as a result of incentive plans. In recent years, incentive plans have become the center of a raging debate. In *Punished by Rewards,* Alfie Kohn (1999) calls them a "carrot on a stick," claiming that they do not always work as intended. Be that as it may, in healthcare today, incentives are very much a part of the satisfiers used to compensate top executive leaders in healthcare. Incentives should:

- attract and retain required talent;
- achieve defined strategic priorities relating to shared vision;
- enhance the organization's performance climate;
- support changes in business direction;
- reinforce executive leadership and managerial direction;
- encourage collaborative teamwork;
- align programs and investments;
- focus change efforts; and
- reward the right results.

Structured correctly, incentive compensation can be an effective way to communicate vision and strategy throughout the organization, link a performance improvement plan to executive leadership actions, and provide an opportunity to share in the resulting success.

Step 5: Coach and Develop

Top executive leaders have a natural desire to improve both their competence and results, and thereby enhance value creation. To do so, they require three key components:

1. The right goals
2. A link to strategy
3. Continual feedback

Setting top leadership goals means establishing the highest priority performance results desired in the future and then operationalizing the strategy. This step gives the board the opportunity to recalibrate the goals for the CEO, or for the CEO to do the same for his/her direct reports on the leadership team. Recalibration of existing goals typically happens during a semi-annual or quarterly review based on internal and/or external factors affecting goals. This step also involves setting new goals for the next performance cycle. Goals should be based on the executive's role description, should be specific and measurable (in terms of time, quality, quantity, and cost), and should be attainable.

Communication is an important part of the process. Top executives need to know what behaviors or competencies they are expected to exhibit, what results they are expected to achieve, and how these behaviors and results will be measured. They must feel confident that the target goals and behaviors are realistic, and they must have the resources necessary to influence and control such goals. This means there must be ongoing dialogue between the board, CEO, and leadership team. The process of goal setting should be mutual. The stronger the concurrence on related expectations, the greater the trust in the system and/or performance assessment process.

Any performance assessment process will fail or succeed depending on strategic links. As goals are set and/or recalibrated for the executive, they must be aligned to the values, culture, vision, and mission. The goals must also effectively cascade downward throughout the organization and thereby link strategic thinking and performance accountability.

Feedback is a critical success factor to the performance assessment process. For feedback to be successful, it must be:

- *actionable:* focused on competencies and results;
- *balanced:* not just negative;
- *based in facts:* not in snap judgments;
- *descriptive:* not vague;
- *non-judgmental:* unbiased and objective; and
- *fair and accurate:* not exaggerated.

To be effective, feedback must also:

- focus on and describe specific performance issues;
- occur close to the performance event;
- reinforce effective performance;
- correct problems;
- suggest choices instead of giving orders;
- talk about the behavior, not the person;
- show appreciation for performance improvements; and
- describe the impact on you (assessor), the leadership team, and the organization.

Usually, the board has the most direct input or feedback to the CEO and indirectly to the other top executive leaders. The top leadership may also receive feedback directly or indirectly and usually informally (i.e., not through a formal "appraisal" process) from medical staff, physician leadership, peers, vendors, suppliers, and/or customers.

In recent years, the popularity of 360-degree and/or upward feedback has increased dramatically in healthcare organizations. As Walter Turnow and Manuel London (1998) explain, in 360-degree feedback, a person's performance is rated by a range of coworkers including supervisors, peers, subordinates, and occasionally customers. Upward feedback is similar, but this comes only from subordinates (usually direct reports) and, occasionally, customers. Both kinds of multisource assessment are considered to be more credible than a single-source assessment, and, therefore, are more likely to influence behavior change. Single source assessment can lead to a misuse of management power.

In addition, multisource assessment has a much stronger interrater reliability, and a strong sense of fairness and balance because employees have an opportunity to influence the behavior of others through feedback. Multisource assessment offers the following advantages:

- *Fair:* less rating inflation, less adverse effect on diversity
- *Accurate:* less bias and more balance
- *Credible:* broader perspective (multiple ratings)
- *Valuable:* more specific feedback and greater performance distinctions
- *Motivational:* more constructive change (peer encouragement)

Typically, specific feedback results are reported directly to the executive(s) and compared with self-ratings. Then the executives confer with those at the next level up (the senior manager with the CEO, or the CEO with the board), to set developmental goals, which are sometimes attached to succession planning, promotion, and pay raises (Tornow and London 1998).

Multisource assessments can also be used as a monitoring tool, to select high-potential individuals, to communicate directly or indirectly what new skills are needed to support strategy, and to help individuals who cannot or will not communicate feedback directly. More and more healthcare organizations are involving customers to participate in multisource assessments to ensure their needs, expectations, and priorities are met. These assessments are used to define performance expectations, reinforce and focus the importance of customer requirements and "competitive advantage," and provide the opportunity to shape performance to changing customer requirements.

CONCLUSION

As Renaissance philosopher Francis Bacon writes in *Of Innovations,* "He who will not apply new remedies must expect new evils—for time is the greatest innovator." Healthcare organizations today confront many difficult challenges and exciting opportunities— all in the context of rapid change. With such high stakes and difficult conditions, top executive leaders have their work cut out for them. They must be able to identify and clarify core values, articulate and communicate the vision and mission, establish strategic goals, and manage change.

Such onerous responsibility must be matched with equally heavy accountability. This requires a rigorous performance assessment process. To ensure effective leadership, evaluators need to establish a continuous process to connect the behavioral attributes of leaders to the results they achieve—aligning leaders' competencies to "outputs" as revealed in key performance indicators.

With this process, evaluators set key performance indicators through many useful tools and methodologies. More importantly, they also create further value through timely and constructive feedback and guidance. The ultimate result is a performance management system that can stand the test of changing times.

REFERENCES

Abrahams, J. 1999. *The Mission Statement Book: 301 Corporate Mission Statements from America's Top Companies.* Berkeley, CA: Ten Speed Press.

American College of Healthcare Executives and American Hospital Association. 1993. *Evaluating the Performance of the Hospital CEO in a Total Quality Management Environment.* Chicago: ACHE.

American College of Healthcare Executives, American Hospital Association, American Medical Association, and Ernst & Young. 1996. *The Partnership Study: A Study of the Roles and Working Relationships of the Hospital Board Chairman, CEO, and Medical Staff President; Executive Summary.* Chicago: ACHE.

Bennis, W. 1989. *On Becoming a Leader.* Reading, MA: Addison-Wesley.

Burgelman, R. A. and Y. L. Doz. 2001. "The Power of Strategic Integration." *MIT Sloan Management Review.* 42 (43): 28–38.

Covey, S. 1989. *The Seven Habits of Highly Effective People.* New York: Simon & Schuster.

Fitz-enz, J. 1997. *The 8 Practices of Exceptional Companies.* New York: AMACOM.

Gilbert, T. F. 1996. *Human Competence.* Amherst: HRD Press.

Hawthorne, G. 2000. "Pay for Performance" *Trustee* (July/August): 9–14.

Heifetz, R. A. 1994. *Leadership Without Easy Answers.* Cambridge, MA: The Belknap Press.

Johnson, L. W. 2000. "The Five-Word CFO Job Description." *Healthcare Financial Management* (August): 29–32.

Kaplan, R. S. and Norton, D. P. 2001. *The Strategy-Focused Organization.* Boston: Harvard Business School Press.

Kohn, A. 1999. *Punished By Rewards: The Trouble with Gold Stars, Incentive Plans, A's, Praise, and Other Bribes.* New York: Houghton-Mifflin.

Lawler, E. E. 2000. *Rewarding Excellence.* San Francisco: Jossey-Bass.

Lawler, E. E. and S. A. Mohrman. 1998. *Strategies for High Performance Organizations—The CEO Report.* San Francisco: Jossey-Bass.

McClellan, D. 1976. *A Guide to Job Competence Assessment.* Boston: McBer.

Moxley, R. S. 2000. *Leadership and Spirit.* San Francisco: Jossey-Bass.

Nanus, B. 1989. *The Leader's Edge: The Seven Keys to Leadership in a Turbulent World.* Chicago: Contemporary Books.

Nanus, B. 1992. *Visionary Leadership.* San Francisco: Jossey-Bass.

Newman, J. F., J. M. Robinson, L. Tyler, and D. M. Dunbar. 2001. "CEO Performance Appraisal: Review and Recommendations/Practitioner Application." *Journal of Healthcare Management* 46 (1): 21–37.

Ray, P. H. and S. R. Anderson. 2000. *The Cultural Creatives.* New York: Harmony Books.

Raynor, M. E. and J. L. Bower. 2001. "Lead From the Center." *Harvard Business Review* 79 (5): 92–105.

Schein, E. H. 1992. *Organizational Culture and Leadership*. San Francisco: Jossey-Bass.

Schein, E. H. 1999. *The Corporate Culture*. San Francisco: Jossey-Bass.

Senge, P. and C. Goran. 2001. "Innovating Our Way to the Next Industrial Revolution." MIT *Sloan Management Review* 42 (3): 24–40.

Sessa, V. I. and J. J. Taylor. 2000. *Executive Selection, Strategies for Success*. San Francisco: Jossey-Bass.

Spencer, L. M. and S. M. Spencer. 1993. *Competencies at Work*. New York: John Wiley & Sons.

Teal, T. 1996. "The Human Side of Management." *Harvard Business Review* (November–December): 35–46.

Tornow, W. and M. London. 1998. *Maximizing the Value of 360-Degree Feedback: A Process for Successful Individual and Organizational Development*. San Francisco: Jossey-Bass.

Treacy, M. and F. Wiersema. 1995. *The Discipline of Market Leaders*. Reading, MA: Addison-Wesley.

Tyler, J. L. 1994. "The Hospital CEO Performance Evaluation, Survey of Current Status. A Survey of CEOs and Board Chairmen." ACHE Fellowship thesis.

CHAPTER 4

Setting Reasonable Compensation: Minimizing Exposure to "Intermediate Sanctions"

Diane Cornwell and Christine Jha

TODAY'S HEALTHCARE ORGANIZATIONS face tremendous pressure to improve organizational efficiency while reducing costs. At the same time, healthcare employers also confront the need to enhance their salary and benefit packages to attract and retain top talent. To increase productivity while at the same time attracting talent, healthcare organizations commonly offer compensation incentive arrangements for key executives and physicians. While the topic of compensation can cause any CEO heartburn, these incentive arrangements deliver an extra dose of heartache to the tax-exempt, not-for-profit healthcare CEO, given the unique laws that govern tax exemption.

By virtue of being exempt under Section 501(c)(3) of the Internal Revenue Code (IRC), a tax-exempt hospital must at all times be both *organized and operated exclusively for one or more exempt purposes*.[1] An organization is *not* considered to be *operated exclusively* for exempt purposes if its net earnings *inure* in whole or in part to the benefit of a *private shareholder or individual*. The term *private shareholder or individual* is typically defined as those persons who have a personal and private interest in the tax-exempt entity, including an organization's directors (or trustees) and officers. The inurement prohibition is absolute, as the law provides no *de*

95

minimis (minimum) exception. Technically, the IRS may revoke an organization's exempt status if it detects *any* amount of inurement—although, historically, this has not been the approach of the Internal Revenue Service (IRS) in resolving such matters.

The IRS Exempt Organization Handbook, an internal training manual of the IRS, states that

". . . the prohibition of inurement in its simplest terms, means that a private shareholder or individual cannot pocket the organization's funds except for reasonable payment for goods or services."

Inurement involves a transaction in which an individual, by virtue of his/her relationship with the organization, receives an unwarranted financial benefit from the organization. Excessive compensation arrangements (such as those arrangements where the compensation is greater than the fair market value of services rendered) can result in inurement and jeopardize an organization's exempt status.

In addition to the inurement prohibition, the tax-exempt healthcare executive must also be concerned with the "private benefit" doctrine. Although distinct from the inurement prohibition, the private benefit doctrine is based on a broad application of inurement and thus may exist in scenarios that also include instances of inurement. Private benefit, unlike inurement, is not limited to insiders. Rather, private benefit can accrue to anyone who engages in transactions with the organization. Additionally, the private benefit doctrine, unlike the inurement ban, is not absolute; private benefit may be allowed in certain situations if such benefit is "incidental" to the overall public purpose. *Incidental private benefit* results where the private benefit occurs not as a result of the pursuit of a private goal, but rather as a necessary outcome of the pursuit of the public goal. In determining whether private benefit has occurred and the degree to which it has occurred, regulators consider all of the relevant facts and circumstances of the situation—including the proportions involved.

In 1996[2], Congress enacted legislation that potentially affects the compensation arrangements between tax-exempt organizations and certain individuals. Now, the executive must review his/her tax-exempt organization's compensation arrangements in light of IRC Section 4958, or what is commonly referred to as *intermediate sanctions*. The sanctions are called intermediate because they represent a middle ground between revoking the tax-exempt status and ignoring the violation.

INTERMEDIATE SANCTIONS: A HISTORY

Prior to the enactment of intermediate sanctions, the IRS, upon finding cases of abuse (such as excessive compensation), could either revoke the organization's tax-exempt status or overlook the abuse. Over time, both options proved unsatisfactory. Revoking an entity's exempt status failed to punish the individuals involved in the abuse. Instead, revocation punished the organization itself as well as the community that relied on the organization's services while the individuals involved in the abuse were free to practice it elsewhere. Obviously, overlooking a violation did not punish abusers—and in fact permitted the abuse to continue.

In a few cases, the IRS could attempt to punish abuses through a "closing agreement process" by levying a penalty on the organization in the closing agreement. Once again, however, the individuals who engaged in the abuse often went unpunished.

On July 30, 1996, President Clinton signed into law the Taxpayer Bill of Rights 2 ("TBOR 2"), which contained provisions referred to as intermediate sanctions. These provisions arose out of growing public perception that powerful individuals associated with charitable, tax-exempt organizations were unfairly exploiting the organizations' status by misusing the organizations' assets to their gain. Imposing sanctions provided the IRS with a more effective (and less extreme) approach for penalizing wrongdoing than revoking tax-exempt status.

In addition, the intermediate sanctions offered a way to raise revenues to offset the cost of the tax cuts contained in TBOR 2.

A few landmark regulatory events are worth noting. In August 1998, the U. S. Treasury Department released proposed regulations that attempted to provide additional guidance with respect to the new intermediate sanctions legislation. Then, after an extended comment period, in January 2001, the U.S. Department of Treasury published temporary regulations.3 A year later, January 2002, the U.S. Department of Treasury removed the temporary regulations and published the final regulations pertaining to intermediate sanctions. At the time of this writing, the final regulations constitute the most authoritative source of guidance for avoiding intermediate sanctions, since the courts have not yet heard and settled an intermediate sanctions case.4 Further guidance may be forthcoming. We can infer from past remarks made by IRS officials that the IRS is developing cases that may result in the imposition of intermediate sanctions. In a panel discussion of the ABA tax section meeting, a senior IRS litigation attorney stated that "Every [Sec.] 4958 matter is being closely monitored and coordinated with the [IRS] national office on both the technical and the counsel side." Directors and officers of healthcare organizations, as well as their advisors, would be wise to keep a close watch on such developments.

Mechanics of Intermediate Sanctions: Key Questions

When planning or documenting a transaction, there are a few questions that must be answered in light of intermediate sanctions.

Are individuals associated with this organization potentially subject to intermediate sanctions?

Intermediate sanctions apply to individuals associated with all entities organized under IRC Sections 501(c)(3)5 and 501(c)(4)6, excluding private foundations. Private foundations are subject to "self-dealing" restrictions, a subject beyond the scope of this chapter.

Furthermore, the regulations specifically exclude certain tax-exempt governmental entities from intermediate sanctions. This exclusion extends to governmental units or affiliates that are either:

- exempt from (or not subject to) taxation without regard to IRC Section 501(a) or
- not required to file an annual Federal return pursuant to Treas. Reg. §1.6033-2(g)(6).

The income of a state institution (i.e., state university) is excluded from taxation by IRC Section 115. As such, a state institution would not be subject to intermediate sanctions.

What individuals in this organization may be subject to intermediate sanctions?

Intermediate sanctions impose an excise tax on any "disqualified person" who exploits his/her position with the exempt organization to engage in an improper transaction with the organization. These types of transactions, under the law, are referred to as *excess benefit transactions*.

In general, a *disqualified person* is any individual who is in a position to exercise substantial influence over the affairs of the organization at any time for five years before an excess benefit transaction occurs. According to the regulations, a disqualified person is defined as:

- Any individual who has substantial influence over the affairs of the organization, such as a president, chief executive officer (CEO), chief financial officer (CFO), chief operating officer (COO), treasurer, or governing board member.
- Any individual who holds powers similar to those of a president, CEO, CFO, COO, treasurer, or governing body member.

- Family members of the individual in a position to exercise substantial influence.
- Certain entities that are controlled by the individual (with 35 percent as the ownership threshold).

What kinds of transactions are considered to be excess benefit transactions?

In order for intermediate sanctions to apply, there must be an "excess benefit transaction" between the organization and a disqualified person. In general, an *excess benefit transaction* is any transaction in which the value of the economic benefit provided by an organization to a disqualified person exceeds the value of the consideration received by the organization in return.

In other words, an excess benefit transaction results when the organization does not deal with the disqualified person on an arm's-length basis. Examples of excess benefits transactions include excessive compensation arrangements and property transactions that are not at fair market value (where the disqualified person buys something from the organization at a fee below market value, or sells or provides something to the organization for a fee above market value).

What happens if there is an excess benefit transaction?

Intermediate sanctions impose a two-tier excise tax against any disqualified person engaging in what the IRS considers to be an excess benefit transaction. (The organization itself is not subject to this tax.) The tax is assessed based on the excess benefit derived from the transaction.

The first tier results in a 25 percent tax on the excess benefit received by the disqualified person. Furthermore, the person must correct the transaction, as described later in this chapter (under "Implications for the Disqualified Individual"). If the person does not correct the excess benefit transaction, then he or she must pay a second-tier tax on the excess benefit of an additional 200 percent.

In addition, intermediate sanctions provide a 10 percent excise tax on any "organization manager" who knowingly and willingly participated in the excess benefit transaction. The organization manager's liability is capped at $10,000 per transaction. Generally, an *organization manager* is defined as an officer, director, or trustee of the organization. Such individuals who knowingly approve an improper transaction are liable.

Finally, as discussed in greater detail later, an organization involved in an excess benefit transaction also has exposure to any applicable prohibitions against inurement and/or private benefit.

Is there a way to minimize exposure from intermediate sanctions?

The single most effective method of minimizing exposure from intermediate sanctions is documentation, documentation, and more documentation. An organization must be diligent in documenting the reasonableness of its transactions with disqualified persons.

The burden of proof is on the individual, not on the IRS. In most cases, the IRS does not have to prove that a particular transaction results in an excess benefit. Rather, the disqualified person (or organization manager) must prove that the transaction in question is reasonable. The regulations, however, provide an exception to this rule. Under the "rebuttable presumption of reasonableness," the transaction is deemed to be reasonable or equal to fair market value (unless the IRS can show otherwise) and, thus, no excess benefit is conferred. To shift the burden of proof to the IRS, all three of the following requirements must be met:

1. An independent, authorized body of the organization approves the arrangement as reasonable.
2. The independent, authorized body of the organization obtains and relies on comparable data in granting its approval.

3. The independent, authorized body of the organization adequately and concurrently documents the basis for its decision.

The remainder of this chapter provides further detail on intermediate sanctions, focusing on compensation payments in the tax-exempt healthcare arena.7 To apply the content of this chapter to their own situations, organizations should consult their tax advisors.

DEFINING DISQUALIFIED PERSONS

A disqualified person is any individual who is in a position to exercise substantial influence over the affairs of the organization. An individual is considered to be a disqualified person if that individual was able to exert substantial influence over the organization at any time for five years before the potential transaction.8 Therefore, it is important to understand both an individual's current and prior relationship with the organization before undertaking (or examining) a transaction.

As the key to being a disqualified person is that individual's ability to exert *substantial influence* over the organization, it is important to understand what is meant by this term. The regulations list persons who, by the virtue of their powers and responsibilities or certain interest they hold, are deemed to exercise substantial influence over the affairs of an organization. These persons include presidents, CEOs, CFOs, COOs, treasurers, and voting members of the organization's governing body.

The determination of whether an individual has the ability to exert substantial influence, however, depends not only on the organization's legal and operational structure, but also on facts and circumstances. The determination is based upon the actual power he or she has within the organization and not merely by the individual's title or formal position. For instance, a cardiology department head who controls the department's operating budget, sets department compensation level, and can legally bind the organization, could be viewed as exercising substantial influence. However, a cardiology department head who does not have any such responsibilities presents a different case. Regulators may consider the influence of such an individual to be less than substantial. Conversely, an individual that does not hold the title of a disqualified person but does hold the powers normally associated with such a title would be considered a disqualified person.

Other persons automatically considered disqualified are family members of disqualified persons and certain entities controlled by a disqualified person. In addition, persons with a material financial interest in a hospital's provider-sponsored organization are considered disqualified persons. A provider-sponsored organization provides health services and is operated and owned by a healthcare provider (or group of providers) who hold a major financial interest in the organization and share the financial risk associated with providing the health services.[9]

For this purpose, family members include spouses, brothers, sisters, spouses of brothers and sisters, ancestors (parents, grandparents, great grandparents), children, grandchildren, great grandchildren, and spouses of children, grandchildren, and great grandchildren. Controlled entities include corporations, partnerships, trusts, and estates where the disqualified person has more than 35 percent of the combined voting power, profits interest, or beneficial interest, respectively.

Example 1

Joan is the president of a hospital, recognized as exempt under IRC Section 501(c)(3). The hospital has a foundation, recognized as exempt under IRC Section 501(c)(3). The foundation awards Joan's son, George, a lucrative technology consulting contract. Joan, by virtue of being president of hospital, oversees the operations of the foundation.

Assuming that Joan holds the powers normally associated with the position of president, Joan is a disqualified person with respect to both the hospital and foundation. As such, George is a disqualified person with respect to both the hospital and foundation by virtue of being the son of a disqualified person.[10]

With the exception of the disqualified persons specifically listed in the regulations, the determination of whether an individual exercises substantial influence depends on facts and circumstances. According to the regulations, the following facts and circumstances suggest substantial influence:

- The person founded the organization.
- The person is a substantial contributor to the organization.[11]
- The person's compensation is primarily based on revenues derived from activities of the organization, or of a particular department or function of the organization, which the person controls.
- The person has or shares authority to control or determine a substantial portion of the organization's capital expenditures, operating budget, or compensation for employees.
- The person manages a discrete segment of activity of the organization, which represents a substantial portion of the activities, assets, income, or expenses of the organization as compared to the organization as a whole.
- The person owns a controlling interest (measured by either vote or value) in a corporation, partnership, or trust that is a disqualified person.
- The party is a nonstock organization controlled, directly or indirectly, by one or more disqualified persons.

Conversely, the following factors tend to indicate that an individual does *not* have substantial influence over the organization:

- The person has taken a bona fide vow of poverty as an employee, agent, or on behalf of a religious group.

- The person is an independent contractor whose sole relationship is providing professional services without having the decision-making authority.
- The person's direct supervisor is not a disqualified person.
- The person does not participate in any management decisions affecting the organization as a whole or affecting any segment or activity of the organization that represents a substantial portion of the activities, assets, income, or expenses of the organization, as compared to the organization as a whole.
- Any preferential treatment the person receives based on the size of that person's donation is also offered to all other donors, making a comparable contribution as part of a solicitation intended to attract a substantial number of contributions.

The regulations provide that specific parties are excluded from being disqualified persons. These exclusions include IRC Section 501(c)(3) and certain 501(c)(4) organizations. Additionally, employees other than board or managerial employees who receive economic benefits, either directly or indirectly from the organization, of less than the amount for a "highly compensated employee"[12] are also excluded, provided that the individual is not otherwise a disqualified person.

The following examples, which are based on the regulations, illustrate the concept of a disqualified person.

Example 1

John is a radiologist at a hospital, recognized as exempt under IRC Section 501(c)(3). John instructs staff with respect to the radiology work he conducts, but he does not supervise other hospital employees. Furthermore, he has no managerial authority over the hospital or its operations. John is paid a fixed salary for his services to the hospital. He is, however, eligible for an incentive award based on the revenues of the radiology department. John's income is more than the highly compensated employee amount. He is not related to any other disqualified person. Furthermore, John does not sit on the governing body of the hospital nor is he an officer of the hospital. The hospital participates in a provider-sponsored organization; however, John does not have a material financial interest in that organization.

Whether John is a disqualified person is a facts and circumstances test. John's compensation is not based primarily on revenues derived from activities of the hospital that he controls. John does not participate in any management decisions impacting the hospital or a discrete segment of the hospital that represents a substantial portion of its activities, assets, income or expenses. Therefore, under these specific facts, John does not have substantial influence over the affairs of the hospital and, accordingly, is not a disqualified person with respect to the hospital.

Example 2

Jill, a cardiologist, is head of the cardiology department of a hospital, an IRC Section 501(c)(3) organization. This department is a major source of patient admissions for the hospital and consequently represents a substantial portion of the hospital's income, relative to the hospital's aggregate income. Jill does not serve on the hospital's governing board nor is she an officer of the hospital. Jill does not have a material financial interest in the provider-organization in which the hospital participates. Jill's compensation package includes salary, retirement and welfare benefits, which is fixed by a three-year renewable employment contract with the hospital. Jill's compensation is higher than the amount referenced for highly compensated individuals.

Whether Jill is a disqualified person is a facts and circumstances test. As head of the department, Jill manages the cardiology department and has authority to allocate budget for the department, which includes authority to distribute incentive bonuses according to criteria set by Jill. Jill's management of a discrete segment of the hospital that represents a substantial portion of its income and activities places Jill in a position to exercise substantial influence over the affairs of the hospital. Under these facts and circumstances, the IRS in the regulations concludes that Jill is a disqualified person with respect to the hospital.

DEFINING AN EXCESS BENEFIT TRANSACTION

To fall within the purview of intermediate sanctions, a disqualified person must engage in an excess benefit transaction with an IRC Section 501(c)(3) or 501(c)(4) organization. An excess benefit transaction is any transaction in which an IRC Section 501(c)(3) or 501(c)(4) organization provides a benefit to (or for the use of) any disqualified person, and where the value of the economic benefit provided exceeds the value of the consideration (including the performance of services) received for providing the benefit. A potential excess benefit transaction is one in which an employee received compensation in excess of fair market value of the services he or she provided to the organization.

To determine if an excess benefit transaction has occurred, one must look at all the consideration and benefits exchanged between the disqualified person and the tax-exempt organization and all entities that are controlled by the tax-exempt organization.[13] For example, in determining the economic benefits conferred to the CEO of a hospital, it is important to consider the benefits provided to the CEO by the hospital's related organizations (i.e., foundation, taxable subsidiary, etc.).

Excess benefit transactions also include indirect transactions whereby an organization transfers economic benefits indirectly (through a controlled subsidiary or intermediary) to a disqualified person. Suppose an organization, under a verbal or written arrangement, provides economic benefits to a third party (intermediary) that in turn provides economic benefits to the disqualified person of the organization. The IRS would examine such an arrangement as a potential excess benefit transaction.

If a tax-exempt organization and a person who is not yet "disqualified" enter into a contract with fixed payments (or another objective formula for determining payment), those payments are not subject to scrutiny under intermediate sanctions—even if the person later becomes disqualified. This is called the "initial contract exception." However, if the contract allows for discretionary payments at some future time, and the person later becomes a disqualified person, then payments received under the contract no longer meet this exception and should be re-examined carefully.

In determining whether an excess benefit transaction has occurred in the compensation context, certain economic benefits may be disregarded. Generally, nontaxable fringe benefits (economic benefits excluded from income under IRC Section 132) and reimbursed expenses under an IRC Section 62 accountable plan are disregarded for intermediate sanctions purposes.

In determining whether compensation is reasonable, regulators do not consider payments or benefits:

- To a volunteer for the organization if the benefit is provided to the general public in exchange for a membership fee or contribution of $75 or less per year.
- To a member of an organization solely on account of the payment of a membership fee.
- To a donor solely on account of a contribution deductible under section 170 (regardless of whether the donor is eligible to claim the deduction).
- To a person solely as member of a charitable class that the applicable tax-exempt organization intends to benefit as part of the accomplishment of the organization's exempt purpose.
- To (or for the use of) a governmental unit defined in Section 170(c)(1), if the payment or benefit is for exclusively public purposes.

Example 1

Sheila is chief operating officer of a hospital exempt under IRC Section 501(c)(3). Assuming that Sheila holds the powers normally associated with such a position, she is a disqualified person with respect to the hospital. As part of its preventive health program, the hospital offers weekly free blood pressure screening to the community at-large. Sheila participates in the screening program. In determining whether Sheila's compensation package is reasonable for intermediate sanctions purposes, the cost of the blood pressure screening is excluded as an IRC 132 nontaxable fringe benefit.

Example 2

Pat is a board member of a hospital exempt under IRC Section 501(c)(3) and, as such, is a disqualified person with respect to the hospital. The hospital controls a supporting foundation, an organization also exempt under IRC Section 501(c)(3). The foundation has an annual fundraising golf tournament, in which each donor giving $50 receives a digital thermometer. In addition to volunteering his time at the tournament, Pat donates $50 and receives the thermometer. In determining whether Pat's compensation package is reasonable for intermediate sanctions purposes, the cost of the digital thermometer is excluded since the benefit (i.e., thermometer) is provided to the general public in exchange for a donation of $75 of less.

REASONABLE COMPENSATION AND EXCESS BENEFIT

An individual's compensation is deemed to be reasonable for the purposes of intermediate sanctions if the value of services is the amount that would ordinarily be paid for like services by like enterprises under like circumstances. The determination of whether compensation is reasonable always depends on the facts and circumstances, including the nature of the services and the organization's operations. Historically, the IRS and the courts considered several factors in determining reasonableness, including:

- Nature, extent, and scope of individual's work
- Character and amount of responsibility of the individual
- Individual's background
- Individual's knowledge of the business
- Size and complexity of business
- Prevailing economic conditions
- Salary scale in the industry
- Availability of fringe benefits
- Individual's contribution to the success of the business

In determining whether an individual's compensation is reasonable for intermediate sanctions purposes, all economic benefits provided by the organization in exchange for the performance of services should be included. The regulations provide the following nonexclusive list of benefits that should be included for purposes of determining the reasonableness of compensation:

- All forms of cash and noncash compensation, including salary, fees, bonuses, severance payments, and deferred and noncash compensation
- Payment of liability insurance premiums for—or reimbursement of—any penalty, tax, or expense of correction owed under intermediate sanctions (unless excludable as a *de minimis* fringe benefit)
- Any expense not reasonably incurred by the person in connection with a civil judicial or administrative proceeding arising out of the person's performance of services on behalf of the organization

- Any expense resulting from an act (or failure to act) where the person has acted wilfully and without reasonable cause
- All other compensatory benefits, whether or not included in gross income for income tax purposes, including payments to welfare benefit plans, both taxable and nontaxable fringe benefits (excluding IRC Section 132 fringe benefits and expense reimbursements under an IRC Section 62 accountable plan) and the economic benefit of a below-market loan

Common fringe benefits that need to be taken into account include:

- Automobiles
- Awards or prizes
- Bonuses
- Cellular telephones
- Club memberships/dues
- Educational/tuition assistance
- Housing allowances
- Insurance
- Meals
- Moving Expenses
- Parking
- Scholarships/fellowships
- Subsidized dining

Example 1

Janice is the CEO of a hospital, an IRC Section 501(c)(3) organization. Her annual salary package is $1,000,000. Comparable salary surveys show the fair market value of Janice's services is $600,000 per year. The IRS could assert that Janice is a disqualified person because she exerts substantial influence as CEO, and that she receives an excess benefit of $400,000 for that service.

Example 2

Robert is CEO of a hospital, an IRC Section 501(c)(3) organization. The hospital has a tax-exempt controlled clinic. As CEO, Robert is responsible for overseeing the activities of the hospital. Robert's duties as CEO make him a disqualified person with respect to the hospital. Robert's compensation package represents the maximum reasonable compensation for his services as CEO. Therefore, any additional economic benefits Robert receives from the hospital without providing additional consideration would constitute an excess benefit transaction. The clinic contracts with Robert to provide certain consulting services, but the contract does not require Robert to perform any additional services for the clinic that he is not already obligated to perform as the hospital's CEO. Therefore, any payment made by the clinic to Robert under the contract represents an indirect excess benefit that the hospital has provided via its controlled entity (the clinic), even if it is paid through the entity and reported as such.

Example 3

A hospital, exempt under IRC Section 501(c)(3), has a wholly-owned taxable subsidiary. Janice, as the CEO of the hospital, is a disqualified person with respect to the hospital. The hospital pays Janice an annual salary of $1,000,000 and reports the amount as compensation for that year. Janice, however, only worked eight months at the hospital and four months at the subsidiary. Taking into account all of the economic benefits the hospital provided to Janice—as well as all the services Janice provided to both the hospital and the subsidiary—the $1,000,000 does not exceed the fair market value of the services Janice performed for the hospital and the subsidiary during the year. As such, under these facts, the hospital does not provide an excess benefit to Janice directly or indirectly.

Example 4

A hospital, an IRC Section 501(c)(3) organization, has a wholly owned taxable subsidiary. Mark is the CEO of the taxable subsidiary and receives salary and benefits for these duties. Mark serves as a voting member of the governing body of the taxable subsidiary. As such, Mark is a disqualified person with regard to the hospital. The hospital provides Mark with compensation for serving on the hospital's governing body, which represents reasonable compensation for the services he provides directly to the hospital as a member of its governing body. Mark's total compensation—his compensation package from the taxable subsidiary and his compensation from the hospital—exceeds reasonable compensation for his services provided to both the hospital and taxable subsidiary collectively. Therefore, the portion of total compensation that exceeds reasonable compensation is an excess benefit provided to Mark.

Example 5

Melanie is a disqualified person who was last employed three years ago by a hospital, an IRC Section 501(c)(3) organization, in a position of substantial influence. The hospital makes a grant to an organization engaged in scientific research. The research organization, which is unrelated to both Melanie and the hospital, advertises for qualified candidates for the research position. Melanie is among several highly qualified candidates who apply for the research position and is hired for the job. Although the hospital provided economic benefits to the research organization, and in connection with the receipt of such benefits, the research organization will provide economic benefits to or for the use of Melanie, the research organization acted with significant business purpose or exempt purpose of its own. There was no evidence of an oral or written agreement or understanding with the hospital and research organization that the grant would be used to provide economic benefits to or for the use of Melanie. Under these specific facts and circumstances, the hospital did not provide an economic benefit directly or indirectly through the use of an intermediary.

Example 6

Susan is hired by a hospital, exempt under IRC Section 501(c)(3), to conduct scientific research. On January 1, 2000, Susan entered into a three-year written employment contract with the hospital. Under the contract terms, Susan is required to work full-time at the hospital's laboratory for a fixed annual salary of $90,000. Immediately prior to entering into the employment contract, Susan was not a disqualified person nor did she become a disqualified person pursuant to the initial contract. However, two years after joining the hospital, Susan marries Chris, who is the child of the hospital's president. As Chris's spouse, Susan is a disqualified person with respect to the hospital. Nonetheless, intermediate sanctions do not apply to the hospital's salary payments to Susan due to the initial contract exception.

Example 7

The facts are the same as above, except that after Susan's marriage to Chris, Susan works only sporadically at the laboratory, and performs no other services for the hospital. Notwithstanding that Susan fails to perform substantially all of her obligations under the initial employment contract, the hospital does not exercise its right to terminate the contract for nonperformance and continues to pay Susan her full salary. Under these specific facts, the IRS in the regulations concluded that Susan received excess compensation: the initial contract exception does not apply to any payments made pursuant to the initial contract during any taxable year in which Susan fails to perform substantially all of her obligations under the initial employment contract.

Implications of an Excess Benefit Transaction

Excess benefit transactions have wide-ranging implications—to the organization, to the disqualified person, and to managers.

Implications for the Organization

Although intermediate sanctions do not result in a tax on the organization, they do stem from an initial finding of either inurement and/or private benefit, which in turn can jeopardize an organization's tax-exempt status. In other words, an excess benefit transaction is not mutually exclusive from inurement and/or private benefit. The intent of intermediate sanctions was to punish those individuals who unfairly exploited an organization's assets for personal gain. The intermediate sanctions legislation, however, was not intended to replace the inurement prohibition or private benefit doctrine. Rather, it was intended to supplement them. If the IRS deems an excess benefit transaction to be egregious, it can still revoke the organization's tax-exempt status. Therefore, an organization should be very diligent in documenting the appropriateness and reasonableness of its transactions.

An organization does have a reporting responsibility with regard to intermediate sanctions. If an excess benefit transaction occurs, the organization must make such a disclosure on its annual Form 990, *Return of Organization Exempt From Income Tax*. Form 990, which is open to the public, requires the organization to describe the type of transaction, identify by name the disqualified person(s) involved, and state whether the transaction was corrected. The information return also requires the organization to disclose the amount of intermediate sanctions tax paid by the disqualified person. This disclosure begins the statute of limitations—the period in which the IRS can assess taxes.

Implications for the Disqualified Person

Excise taxes are assessed against any disqualified person who engages in an excess benefit transaction. As stated earlier, the tax, which is two-tiered, is calculated on the excess benefit derived from the transaction. First, a 25 percent tax is assessed on the excess benefit (the amount of payment exceeding the fair market value of the consideration). If the excess benefit is corrected within prescribed time periods and it can be established that the transaction was due to reasonable cause and not willful neglect, the first-tier tax will not be levied. If the disqualified person has already paid the tax in the above situation, then there may be an opportunity for a refund. If the excess benefit is not corrected within a prescribed time, the IRS will assess an additional tax equal to 200 percent of the excess benefit.

In order to correct an excess benefit transaction, the transaction must be undone so that the financial position of the organization is restored to a state no worse than it was in before the transaction occurred. The regulations provide specific types of acceptable forms of correction, which include making cash payments to the organization and returning the specific property involved in the transaction. Additionally, the disqualified person is assessed interest on the excess benefit for the period from the date the transaction occurred to the date of correction.

Example 1

Melinda is treasurer of a hospital foundation. As treasurer, she has authority over authorizing payments on behalf of the foundation. Melinda receives a $500,000 bonus. It is later determined that the bonus is an excess benefit conferred upon Melinda. Melinda does not correct the excess benefit. As such, Melinda is initially at risk for $125,000 in first-tier excise taxes ($500,000 excess benefit times 25 percent first-tier tax) plus restoration of the excess benefit amount and interest.

If Melinda does not take corrective action, she would be at risk for the second-tier taxes as well. Her second-tier tax liability could be $1 million ($500,000 excess benefit times 200 percent second tier tax). Melinda's total tax liability could be $1.25 million.

Example 2

Marvin is COO of a hospital. The hospital hires an advertising firm owned by Marvin's brother, Brian. Brian is considered a disqualified person. Brian's firm is paid $300,000 for the services. The IRS subsequently determines that Brian received an excess benefit of $60,000, as the fair market value of his firm's advertising services is $240,000. The IRS assesses Brian $15,000 ($60,000 excess benefit times 25 percent first-tier tax), plus restoration of the excess benefit and interest.

Brian does not repay the hospital the excess benefit, nor does he take any other further corrective action. Accordingly, the IRS assesses Brian an additional tax of $120,000 ($60,000 excess benefit times 200 percent second-tier tax). Brian's total tax liability is now $135,000 ($15,000 first tier plus $120,000 second-tier taxes).

The above examples are for illustrative purposes only. It is unlikely that anyone, upon being named as a participant in an excess benefit transaction, would fail to correct the transaction in order to avoid the second-tier tax.

Implications for Organization Managers

Intermediate sanctions also result in a separate tax on organization managers who knowingly participate in excess benefit transactions, regardless of whether such individual personally benefited from the transaction. Organization managers are generally officers, directors, and trustees. This penalty tax is equal to 10 percent of the excess benefit amount, but limited to $10,000 per excess benefit transaction. The tax is assessed only if the manager's actions were willful and without reasonable cause. If the IRS finds that more than one organization manager authorized or participated in the transaction, then all of them are jointly and severally liable for the tax.

The regulations provide a safe harbor for organization managers who sought and followed expert professional advice on a transaction that was later determined to be an excess benefit transaction. In such circumstance, the organization manager will not be assessed the tax. To qualify for this safe harbor, the manager must have fully disclosed the factual situation to the professional and relied on advice from that professional in a reasoned written opinion that the transaction did not constitute an excess benefit transaction. Expert professionals specifically cited in the regulations include legal counsel (including in-house counsel), certified public accountants or accounting firms with expertise regarding the relevant tax matters, and certain independent valuation experts.

Example 1

John is a board member of a tax-exempt hospital and approved Joan's $1,200,000 annual compensation package. The IRS later determined that the fair market value of Joan's services was $900,000. John, an organization manager under the law, approved the transaction. The IRS could assess John $10,000 in tax (the organization manager's tax is 10 percent of the excess benefit, but limited to $10,000 per transaction).

Example 2

William is a board member of a tax-exempt hospital. As a board member, he reviewed and approved the CFO's compensation package based on a written opinion from a law firm that the compensation package did *not* confer an excess benefit to the CFO. It was subsequently determined that the compensation package did confer an excess benefit of $85,000. Based on the fact that William relied on expert advice in making his decision, he will likely not be imposed the 10 percent excise tax applicable to organization managers.

REBUTTABLE PRESUMPTION OF REASONABLENESS

The regulations provide a safe harbor exception referred to as the rebuttable presumption of reasonableness. If the IRS questions the reasonableness of a payment, it is up to the organization and/or disqualified person to prove that the payment was reasonable and the transfer of property occurred at fair market value. However, under the safe harbor exception, the organization can shift the burden of proof requirement to the IRS. In general, this exception provides that under certain conditions (for example, if certain documentation is in place), a transaction may be deemed reasonable unless proven otherwise by the IRS.

To qualify for the safe harbor exception with respect to a particular transaction, *all* of the following three requirements must be met:

1. An independent, authorized body of the organization approved the transaction in advance.
2. The independent, authorized body obtained and relied upon appropriate comparability data prior to making its decision.
3. The independent, authorized body adequately documented

the basis for its determination concurrently with making that determination.

If these three requirements are satisfied, penalty excise taxes could be imposed only if the IRS develops sufficient contrary evidence to demonstrate that an excess benefit transaction occurred.

Meeting the First "Rebuttable Presumption" Test

The first test requires that an independent, *authorized body* of the organization approve the transaction. The regulations defines an authorized body as:

- The governing body (i.e., the board of directors, board of trustees, or equivalent controlling body) of the organization;
- A committee of the governing body, which may be composed of any individuals permitted under State law to serve on such a committee, to the extent that the committee is permitted by the State law to act on behalf of the governing body; or
- To the extent permitted under State law, other parties authorized by the governing body of the organization to act on its behalf by following procedures specified by the governing body in approving compensation arrangements or property transfers.

To be deemed independent, the body must be composed of individuals who do not have a conflict of interest with respect to the transaction under review. The regulations provide a list of circumstances that indicate that an authorized body does not have a conflict of interest with respect to a transaction:

- No member of the authorized body is deemed to be a disqualified person or is a relative of any disqualified person.

- No member of the authorized body is in an employment relationship subject to the direction or control of any disqualified person involved in the transaction.
- No member of the authorized body received compensation or other payment subject to approval by any disqualified person participating in or benefiting from the transaction.
- No member of the authorized body has a financial interest affected by the transaction.
- No disqualified person has approved or will approve a transaction providing economic benefits to any member of the authorized body approving the transaction.

As conflicts of interest are not always obvious, especially in organizations with a complex organizational structure, it may be advantageous for an organization to implement a conflict of interest policy. Such a policy is an important mechanism to ensure that the organization is operating for the benefit of the community. The policy should apply to any interested person, such as trustees and principal officers. The IRS developed a model conflicts-of-interest policy for tax-exempt organizations as a means by which the organization could ensure that related party transactions were reviewed by an independent group or board. Although the model policy may not address all issues raised by intermediate sanctions law, it is nonetheless a good resource. For a copy of the model policy, see Appendix 4A at the end of this chapter.

As the model policy indicates, the IRS defines a person with a "financial interest" as any person who directly or indirectly through business, investment, or family has:

- An ownership or investment in any entity with which the tax-exempt organization has a transaction or arrangement.
- A compensation arrangement with the tax-exempt organization or with any entity or individual with which the organization has a transaction or arrangement.
- A potential ownership or investment in, or compensation

arrangement with, any entity or individual with which the tax-exempt organization is negotiating a transaction or arrangement.

The authorized body of the organization may authorize others to act on its behalf in a particular transaction, and those other persons may claim the safe harbor exception for the transaction even though the full authorized body does not vote with respect to the transactions. The persons delegated the responsibility are viewed as organization managers for purposes of intermediate sanctions with respect to the transaction approved.

Meeting the Second "Rebuttal Presumption" Test

To satisfy the second rebuttable presumption requirement, the authorized body must obtain and rely on appropriate comparability data. The definition provided by the regulations states that this condition is met if, given the knowledge and expertise of its members, the authorized body has information sufficient to determine whether, under intermediate sanctions, the transaction is reasonable. Specifically, in the case of compensation, relevant information includes, but is not limited to:

- Compensation levels paid by similarly situated organizations, both taxable and nontaxable, for functionally comparable positions.
- Current compensation surveys compiled by independent firms.
- Actual written offers from similar institutions competing for the services of the disqualified person.

The regulations provide a safe harbor for smaller organizations (defined as organizations with gross receipts of less than $1 million dollars) with regard to obtaining comparable data. Such organizations may meet the safe harbor by collecting comparable data for three similar positions in similar communities. For larger organizations, however, the regulations do not specify the amount of comparable data or sources needed to satisfy this portion of the rebuttable presumption of reasonableness.

Meeting the Third Rebuttable Presumption Test

Under the third requirement, the authorized body must adequately document its decision. The documentation, which may be either written or electronic format, must note the following:

- Terms of the transaction that was approved and the date it was approved
- Members of the authorized body who were present during debate on the transaction that was approved and those who voted on it
- Comparability data obtained and relied upon by the authorized body and how the data was obtained
- Any actions taken with respect to consideration of the transaction by anyone who is otherwise a member of the authorized body but had a conflict of interest with respect to the transaction

If the authorized body claims that reasonable compensation for a transaction is higher or lower than fair market value of the comparability data obtained, then it must record the basis for its determination. To document a decision concurrently, the authorized body must prepare records before the later of the next meeting of the authorized body or within 60 days after the final action or actions of the authorized body are taken.

Records must be reviewed and approved by the authorized body as reasonable, accurate, and complete within a reasonable timeframe thereafter. The authorized body must meet before the organization makes any payments to the disqualified person. If a payment is made without the proper documentation, the rebuttable presumption is not available.

In his article, "Rebuttable Presumption Procedure is Key to Easy Intermediate Sanctions Compliance," the IRS director of exempt organizations includes a rebuttable presumption checklist. Although the article and checklist are not official IRS guidance, the checklist can help organizations document how they have met requirements of the rebuttable presumption. This checklist appears in Appendix 4B.

The following examples, which are based on the regulations, illustrate considerations pertaining to rebuttable presumption of reasonableness.

Example 1

A hospital, defined under IRC Section 501(c)(3), is renewing its employment contracts. Before renewing the contracts of the hospital's CEO and CFO, the hospital's governing board commissioned a customized compensation survey from an independent firm that specializes in consulting on issues related to executive placement and compensation. The survey covered executives with comparable responsibilities at a significant number of taxable and tax-exempt hospitals. The survey data are sorted by a number of different variables, including the size of the hospitals and the nature of the services they provide, the level of experience and specific responsibilities of the executives, and the composition of the annual compensation packages. The board members all received copies of the survey results, along with a detailed written analysis comparing the hospital's executives to those covered by the survey. They also had an opportunity to ask questions of a member of the firm that prepared the survey. Given these facts, the survey, as prepared and presented to hospital's board, constitutes appropriate data as to comparability.

Example 2

The facts are the same as above, except that one year later, the hospital is negotiating a new contract with its CEO. The governing board of the hospital has no information indicating that the relevant market conditions have changed or that the results of the prior year's survey are no longer valid. Therefore, the hospital may continue to rely on the independent compensation survey prepared for the prior year in setting annual compensation under the new contract.

CONCLUSION: LIVING WITH INTERMEDIATE SANCTIONS

For tax-exempt not-for-profit healthcare executives, the key to successfully complying with the intermediate sanctions law is careful planning and documentation of compensation arrangements. When approving existing compensation arrangements, responsible parties should review and document these arrangements carefully, while considering implications of these arrangements in light of the regulations. When an organization is considering implementing new compensation arrangements, it may wish to solicit assistance from professionals (i.e., accountants, valuation experts, and attorneys) in determining the tax ramifications—not only under intermediate sanctions, but also in light of the inurement prohibition, private benefit doctrine, compensation reporting, and Form 990 disclosures.[14]

NOTES

1. The Internal Revenue Code is found in Title 26 of the U.S. Code. All the tax laws can be found in this section. For example, Section 501 (c)(3) is a section of the Code. It is found in 26 U.S.C., Subtitle A, Chapter 1, Subpart F, Part 1,

Section 501. The full text of Section 501 and other sections of the Code may be found at *www.gpo.gov/us/code/title26/title26.html*. All citations in this chapter are taken directly from the Code unless otherwise indicated.

2. The law was enacted on July 30, 1996. However, it is effective for transactions occurring on or after September 14, 1995.

3. The preamble to the temporary regulations explains the changes between the proposed regulations and the temporary regulations. The preamble to the final regulations explains the changes between the temporary regulations and the final regulations.

4. In December 1999, *Tax Analyst* reported the filing of a court case involving the IRS' determination that a conversion of a nontaxable organization into a for-profit entity controlled by disqualified persons resulted in an excess benefit transaction subject to IRC Section 4958.

5. IRC Section 501(c)(3) states "Corporations, and any community chest, fund, or foundation, organized and operated exclusively for religious, charitable, scientific, testing for public safety, literary, or educational purposes, or to foster national or international amateur sports competition (but only if no part of its activities involve the provision of athletic facilities or equipment), or for the prevention of cruelty to children or animals, no part of the net earnings of which inures to the benefit of any private shareholder or individual, no substantial part of the activities of which is carrying on propaganda, or otherwise attempting, to influence legislation (except as otherwise provided in subsection (h), and which does not participate in, or intervene in (including the publishing or distributing of statements), any political campaign on behalf of (or in opposition to) any candidate for public office."

6. IRC Section 501(c)(4) states "Civic leagues or organizations not organized for profit but operated exclusively for the pro-

motion of social welfare, or local associations of employees, the membership of which is limited to the employees of a designated person or persons in a particular municipality, and the net earnings of which are devoted exclusively to charitable, educational, or recreational purposes."

7. This discussion is based on the regulations, which also include various nonhealthcare and noncompensation concepts, examples, and terms not discussed here. Readers should consult the regulations for insight on how intermediate sanctions apply to nonhealthcare exempt organizations as well as to noncompensation related transactions.

8. However, the period may be shorter. The period may begin on September 14, 1995, the effective date of Intermediate Sanctions.

9. Provider-sponsored organization is defined in section 1855(e) of the Social Security Act, 42 U.S.C. 1395w-25.

10. Some examples in this chapter come from the regulations under TBOR 2. In some cases, the author has adapted the examples to the healthcare setting.

11. In determining whether an individual is a substantial contributor, only contributions received by the organization during its current taxable year and the four preceding taxable years are taken into account.

12. The dollar threshold for being a highly compensated employee is adjusted for inflation on an annual basis. For 2002, the threshold is $90,000. Thresholds for the previous years are as follows: 2001–$85,000, 2000–$85,000, 1999–$80,000, 1998–$80,000, 1997–$80,000, 1996–$66,000 and 1995–$66,000.

13. Generally speaking, a controlled entity is one in which the tax-exempt organization has ownership of more than a 50 percent interest.

14. For a guide to Form 990 disclosures, see Chapter 5.

Internal Revenue Service Model Conflicts of Interest Policy (Revised 1999)

ARTICLE I

Purpose

The purpose of the conflicts of interest policy is to protect the Corporation's interest when it is contemplating entering into a transaction or arrangement that might benefit the private interest of an officer or director of the Corporation. This policy is intended to supplement but not replace any applicable state laws governing conflicts of interest applicable to nonprofit and charitable corporations.

ARTICLE II

Definitions

1. Interested Person

Any director, principal officer, or member of a committee with board delegated powers who has a direct or indirect financial interest, as defined below, is an interested person. If a person is an interested person with respect to any entity in the health care system of which the Corporation is a part, he or she is an interested person with respect to all entities in the health care system.

2. Financial Interest

A person has a financial interest if the person has, directly or indirectly, through business, investment or family—

a. an ownership or investment interest in any entity with which the Corporation has a transaction or arrangement, or
b. a compensation arrangement with the Corporation or with any entity or individual with which the Corporation has a transaction or arrangement, or
c. a potential ownership or investment interest in, or compensation arrangement with, any entity or individual with which the Corporation is negotiating a transaction or arrangement.

Compensation includes direct and indirect remuneration as well as gifts or favors that are substantial in nature.

A financial interest is not necessarily a conflict of interest. Under Article III, *Section 2,* a person who has a financial interest may have a conflict of interest only if the appropriate board or committee decides that a conflict of interest exists.

ARTICLE III

Procedures

1. Duty to Disclose

In connection with any actual or possible conflicts of interest, an interested person must disclose the existence of his or her financial interest and must be given the opportunity to disclose all material facts to the directors and members of committees with board delegated powers considering the proposed transaction or arrangement.

2. Determining Whether a Conflict of Interest Exists

After disclosure of the financial interest and all material facts, and after any discussion with the interested person, he/she shall leave the board or committee meeting while the determination of a conflict of interest is discussed and voted upon. The remaining board or committee members shall decide if a conflict of interest exists.

3. Procedures for Addressing the Conflict of Interest

a. An interested person may make a presentation at the board or committee meeting, but after such presentation, he/she shall leave the meeting during the discussion of, and the vote on, the transaction or arrangement that results in the conflict of interest.

b. The chairperson of the board or committee shall, if appropriate, appoint a disinterested person or committee to investigate alternatives to the proposed transaction or arrangement.

c. After exercising due diligence, the board or committee shall determine whether the Corporation can obtain a more advantageous transaction or arrangement with reasonable efforts from a person or entity that would not give rise to a conflict of interest.

d. If a more advantageous transaction or arrangement is not reasonably attainable under circumstances that would not give rise to a conflict of interest, the board or committee shall determine by a majority vote of the disinterested directors whether the transaction or arrangement is in the Corporation's best interest and for its own benefit and whether the transaction is fair and reasonable to the Corporation and shall make its decision as to whether to enter into the transaction or arrangement in conformity with such determination.

4. Violations of the Conflicts of Interest Policy

a. If the board or committee has reasonable cause to believe that a member has failed to disclose actual or possible conflicts of interest, it shall inform the member of the basis for such belief and afford the member an opportunity to explain the alleged failure to disclose.

b. If, after hearing the response of the member and making such further investigation as may be warranted in the circumstances, the board or committee determines that the member has in fact failed to disclose an actual or possible conflict of interest, it shall take appropriate disciplinary and corrective action.

ARTICLE IV

Records of Proceedings

The minutes of the board and all committee with board-delegated powers shall contain—

1. the names of the persons who disclosed or otherwise were found to have a financial interest in connection with an actual or possible conflict of interest, the nature of the financial interest, any action taken to determine whether a conflict of interest was present, and the board's or committee's decision as to whether a conflict of interest in fact existed.

2. the names of the persons who were present for discussions and votes relating to the transaction or arrangement, the content of the discussion, including any alternatives to the proposed transaction or arrangement, and a record of any votes taken in connection therewith.

ARTICLE V

Compensation

1. A voting member of the board of directors who receives compensation, directly or indirectly, from the Corporation for services is precluded from voting on matters pertaining to that member's compensation.
2. A physician who is a voting member of the board of directors and receives compensation, directly or indirectly, from the Corporation for services is precluded from discussing and voting on matters pertaining to that member's and other physicians' compensation. No physician or physician director, either individually or collectively, is prohibited from providing information to the board of directors regarding physician compensation.
3. A voting member of any committee whose jurisdiction includes compensation matters and who receives compensation, directly or indirectly, from the Corporation for services is precluded from voting on matters pertaining to that member's compensation.
4. Physicians who receive compensation, directly or indirectly, from the Corporation, whether as employees or independent contractors, are precluded from membership on any committee whose jurisdiction includes compensation matters. No physician, either individually or collectively, is prohibited from providing information to any committee regarding physician compensation.

ARTICLE VI

Annual Statements

Each director, principal officer and member of a committee with board delegated powers shall annually sign a statement which affirms that such person—

a. has received a copy of the conflicts of interest policy,
b. has read and understands the policy,
c. has agreed to comply with the policy, and
d. understands that the Corporation is a charitable organization and that in order to maintain its federal tax exemption it must engage primarily in activities which accomplish one or more of its tax-exempt purposes.

ARTICLE VII

Periodic Reviews

To ensure that the Corporation operates in a manner consistent with its charitable purposes and that it does not engage in activities that could jeopardize its status as an organization exempt from federal income tax, periodic reviews shall be conducted. The periodic reviews shall, at a minimum, include the following subjects:

a. Whether compensation arrangements and benefits are reasonable and are the result of arm's-length bargaining.
b. Whether acquisitions of physician practices and other provider services result in inurement or impermissible private benefit.
c. Whether partnership and joint venture arrangements and arrangements with management service organizations and physician hospital organizations conform to written policies, are properly recorded, reflect reasonable payments for goods and services, further the Corporation's charitable purposes and do not result in inurement or impermissible private benefit.
d. Whether agreements to provide health care and agreements with other health care providers, employees, and third party payors further the Corporation's charitable purposes and do not result in inurement or impermissible private benefit.

ARTICLE VIII

Use of Outside Experts

In conducting the periodic reviews provided for in Article VII, the Corporation may, but need not, use outside advisors. If outside experts are used their use shall not relieve the board of its responsibility for ensuring that periodic reviews are conducted.

Rebuttable Presumption Checklist

1. Name of disqualified person: _____
2. Position under consideration: _____
3. Duration of contract (1 yr., 3 yr., etc): _____
   Proposed Compensation:
       Salary: _____
       Bonus: _____
       Deferred compensation: _____
       Fringe benefits (list, excluding Sec. 132 fringes):

       _____

       _____

       Liability insurance premiums: _____
       Foregone interest on loans: _____
       Other: _____
4. Description of types of comparability data relied upon
   (e.g., association survey, phone inquiries, etc.):
       a) _____
       b) _____
       c) _____
       d) _____ etc.
5. Sources and amounts of comparability data:
       Salaries_____
       Bonuses: _____
       Deferred compensation: _____
       Fringe benefits (list, excluding Sec. 132 fringes):

       _____

       _____

       _____

Liability insurance premiums:

_____

Foregone interest on loans: _____
Others: _____
Office or file where comparability data kept: _____
7. Total proposed compensation: _____
8. Maximum total compensation per comparability data:
9. Compensation package approved by authorized body:
    Salary: _____
    Bonus: _____
    Fringe benefits (list, excluding Sec. 132 fringes):

    _____

    Deferred compensation: _____
    Liability insurance premiums: _____
    Foregone interest on loans: _____
    Other: _____
10. Date compensation approved by authorized body:

_____

11. Members of the authorized body present (indicate with X if voted in favor):

_____

_____

_____

12. Comparability data relied upon by approving body and how data was obtained:
13. Names of and actions (if any) by members of authorized body having conflict of interest:
14. Date of preparation of this documentation (must be prepared by the later of next meeting of authorized body, or 60 days after authorized body approved compensation):

_____

15. Date of approval of this documentation by Board (must be within reasonable time after preparation of documentation above):

_____

Created by Steven T. Miller, Director Exempt Organizations, Internal Revnue Service.

Wealth Accumulation Through Income Deferral: A Guide for Healthcare Organizations and Executives

Jeffrey D. Frank, Daniel B. Kennedy, and David D. Scaife

ONE OF THE most important considerations in the design of any executive compensation program is balance—in particular, a balance between the financial goals of executives and the business objectives of organizations. Fortunately, both are achievable, thanks to income deferral as a strategy for wealth accumulation. Of course, this is "easier said than done." Wealth accumulation encompasses a broad range of possible solutions, and involves a number of factors affecting both the executives and their organizations. This chapter explains why and how healthcare organizations help their executives accumulate wealth through deferred compensation, and discusses the most common ways they can do this—qualified and nonqualified plans, insurance-based products, and mutual fund option plans.

BACKGROUND

Wealth accumulation strategies have assumed an increasingly important role in healthcare organizations for the following reasons:

- First, tax-advantaged wealth accumulation strategies represent a significant portion of the total compensation package in companies outside the healthcare sector. Therefore, in order to attract and retain qualified executives, many healthcare organizations have added such plans or enhanced existing ones. This is especially true in not-for-profit (nontaxable) healthcare organizations, which are turning to such plans in order to compete with their for-profit (taxable) peers.
- Second, many organizations have eliminated their defined benefit pension plans, or reduced the benefit levels such plans provide. As a result, these organizations and their executives must provide the tools to enable executives to build a sufficient foundation for their retirement income needs. Deferred compensation plans provide a way to do this.
- Finally, many organizations utilize deferred compensation as a "golden handcuff" to retain executive talent.

For these reasons, income deferral and other wealth accumulation programs should play an integral part of any organization's total compensation strategy and framework.

This chapter provides an overview of income deferral approaches, starting with the economics of the deferral decisions. Next, we review design considerations from the perspective of the potential participants and the employer. These include the financial reporting and tax treatment of each alternative, legal and regulatory considerations, the business objectives of the program, and the financial performance that can be achieved by each of the available solutions in the compensation "toolkit." Finally, we provide a review of the most common deferred income approaches. The choice of the "right" program for any particular situation involves a careful consideration of the features, benefits, and implications of each potential solution.

ECONOMICS

To understand the rationale for income deferral strategies, it is useful to look at an example of the power of pre-tax investing. Based on our training in financial concepts such as the time value of money, most of us would prefer to receive a dollar today rather than at some future point in time. However, it may be advantageous to defer receipt of that dollar and avoid the associated taxation if we can invest the money on a pre-tax basis and withdraw the proceeds at a later time. This is the basic premise of most retirement plans, including qualified pension plans, 401(k) plans, 403(b) plans, and many forms of nonqualified retirement programs. These plans can be especially beneficial if beneficiaries invest their assets in competitive investments over a long period of time.

To illustrate this point, let us assume the following facts:

- An executive is eligible for a bonus of $10,000 on December 31, 2001.
- Tax rates for this individual are 36 percent for federal income tax, 0 percent for state income tax, and 20 percent for long-term capital gains, remaining unchanged over the time periods in this example.
- The executive chooses a diversified mutual fund that will result in annual appreciation of 9 percent over the time periods in this example.

The executive can choose between the following:

- Take receipt of the $10,000 bonus on December 31, 2001, and pay ordinary income tax; invest the net proceeds and sell the entire balance at the end of the investment period (from 5 to 30 years in our example); or
- Defer receipt of the $10,000 bonus and invest the entire amount in the mutual fund on a pre-tax basis for the investment period (from 5 years to 30 years in our example), and sell the entire balance at the end of the investment period.

Table 5.1 and Figure 5.1 summarize the rest of this analysis.

Each of the assumptions above has an important influence on the financial modeling in this example. The deferral election may be even more advantageous if the executive can delay the receipt of the compensation beyond the date of retirement, when the effective tax rates will be even lower. However, other factors may reduce the advantage of the deferral election, such as a reduction in capital gains tax rates.

While the income deferral strategy yields a significant improvement over the after-tax investment, such an election is not always a clear-cut choice. The section below discusses issues to be considered, for both the organization and the potential participants in these plans.

DESIGN CONSIDERATIONS

As mentioned earlier, it is important to balance the participants' financial goals with the organization's business objectives. To achieve and maintain this balance means considering a broad range of compensation program alternatives. It also means understanding the precise implications of these alternatives, many of which are highly technical and subject to change as a result of various regulatory and business developments. (It is important to assess the reasonable compensation implications of any arrangement.) Understanding these technicalities can help not only in the planning stage, but also in implementing and monitoring the plans. Key considerations for plan design, implementation, and ongoing monitoring include the following.

Considerations for executives:

- Current income requirements and participation in other plans (i.e., "How much money can I afford to defer?")
- Investment alternatives and financial performance
- Time period of potential deferral

Table 5.1: Deferral vs. Non-deferral: A Comparison of Results

Net Realizable Value as of:	Scenario A (Non-deferral)	Scenario B (Deferral)	Improvement (%)
Year 5	$9,158	$9,847	7.5%
Year 10	$13,401	$15,151	13.1%
Year 15	$19,930	$23,312	17.0%
Year 20	$29,975	$35,868	19.7%
Year 25	$45,430	$55,188	21.5%
Year 30	$69,211	$84,913	22.7%

- Potential tax rate changes and/or changes in applicable tax treatment
- Ability to access account balances (e.g., hardship or elective withdrawals)
- Degree of individual control over date and amount of income recognition
- Security of balances (e.g., potential loss of benefits in a non-qualified plan—explained below)
- Integration with financial and tax planning (e.g., estate plans, portfolio diversification, and death benefits)
- Restrictions included in contracts or agreements

Considerations for the organization:

- Financial accounting treatment
- Cash flow requirements
- Administrative complexity
- Tax treatment, reporting, and withholding
- Supportive alignment with the organization's business strategy and compensation philosophy
- Effect on reasonable compensation reviews
- Ability to structure plans with retention devices (e.g., "golden handcuffs") and performance incentives

Figure 5.1: Advantage of Deferring Income

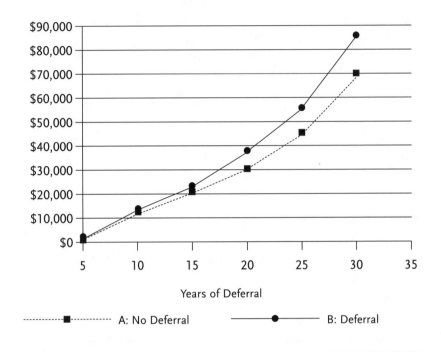

Years of Deferral

---◼--- A: No Deferral   —●— B: Deferral

- Risk of employee attrition and morale problems if plans are not structured appropriately
- Securities law and other legal considerations

In considering these factors, planners must be aware of the natural conflicts between the executives' goals and the organization's objectives. Most executives will want maximum potential compensation with no restrictions, while most organizations will want to maintain at-market, performance-based pay levels while imposing restrictions, such as vesting requirements, payouts contingent on meeting performance goals, and non-compete agreements. To the extent possible, plans should have a flexible structure that will meet the needs of a diverse group of executives, while also protecting the organization from the loss of key executive talent.

To pay what the market will bear (not significantly lower or higher), organizations should benchmark against current pay practices in their employment markets. In doing so, they will need to consider multiple sources of information. One of the challenges in benchmarking pay practices is that many survey sources only include data for a subset of the available programs—cash compensation, employee benefits, or features in deferred compensation plans—but not for a complete package.

COMMON STRATEGIES

Having considered the background and basic economics of wealth accumulation plans, an organization can then select a wealth accumulation approach. The following section provides an overview of several of the most common wealth accumulation strategies.

A wide range of potential wealth accumulation strategies exist, including equity-based pay (e.g., stock options and restricted stock grants), cash-based long-term incentives, supplemental executive retirement plans (SERPs), and various types of deferred compensation plans—the focus of this chapter.

Deferred compensation plans are vehicles for employees to accumulate wealth for the future, either through voluntary deferrals and/or employer contributions. Commonly associated with retirement, deferred compensation arrangements can be designed to address differing goals. For example, they can provide retirement benefits to executives hired in mid-career from another employer, encourage early retirement or retention through a specified period of time, or enable executives to save for their own retirement.

There are two main kinds of retirement plans: qualified and nonqualified. Both enable wealth accumulation through pre-tax appreciation in various assets, but they do vary. This chapter will focus on nonqualified plans. (For a brief primer on qualified plans, see Figure 5.2.)

Figure 5.2: Qualified Retirement Plans: A Primer

A qualified plan is one that meets the requirements of Internal Revenue Code (IRC) Section 401(a), or Section 403(b). This qualification provides the plan with several principal benefits:
- Income earned by the qualified plan is exempt from taxation while plan assets are held in a tax-exempt trust or annuity.
- Assets in the qualified plan are protected from the employer's general creditors.
- Employer contributions to a qualified plan are tax deductible within certain limitations.
- Employer contributions on behalf of its employees are not taxable to employees until the benefits are actually distributed.

Qualified plans consist of two basic types: defined contribution plans and defined benefit plans.
- A defined contribution plan, such as a 401(k) plan, profit sharing plan, and money purchase pension plan, provides an individual account for each participant. Future benefits are based solely on the amount in this account.
- A defined benefit plan is designed to provide a pre-determined level of benefits to an employee after retirement. The most common form of defined benefit plan determines benefits based on the employee's earnings, age, and years of service as of the date of retirement, and these benefits are generally paid for the balance of the employee's life.

The principal drawback of qualified plans is the fact that they are subject to the provisions of the Employee Retirement Income Security Act (ERISA), which contains strict guidelines regarding employee participation and nondiscrimination, funding of plan assets, limitations on deductions, and reporting requirements.

Most executive compensation planning today focuses on non-qualified retirement plans—generally deemed "supplemental" (because they supplement qualified plans). Therefore, the remainder of this chapter will discuss such plans, including traditional forms of qualified deferred compensation plans, insurance-based arrangements, and mutual fund option plans. (Note: There are many variations on the alternatives discussed in this section, and it is important to monitor the ever-changing field of executive compensation for recent developments, rulings, and legislative changes.)

TRADITIONAL FORMS OF NONQUALIFIED DEFERRED COMPENSATION

Qualified deferred compensation plans are a creation of U.S. tax law. Generally cash-based, these plans can include elective deferrals by participants, employer contributions, and earnings on the invested funds. These plans are primarily governed by Internal Revenue Code (IRC) Section 401(a), as explained in Figure 5.2.

Nonqualified plans are arrangements that fail to meet one or more of the requirements for a qualified plan. In not-for-profit (tax-exempt) organizations, nonqualified plans are governed by IRC Section 457, which contains special limitations on the amount of compensation that can be deferred for a plan year and the circumstances under which benefits may be paid under the plan. These limitations are "special" in the sense that they differ from the tax treatment accorded nonqualified deferred plans of for-profit employers. Because so many healthcare institutions operate as not-for-profit charities, we will provide additional details on this important section of tax law.

Section 457(b) prescribes a number of conditions that must be satisfied to treat a nonqualified plan as an "eligible" 457 plan. The most significant requirement of Section 457(b) is that annual deferrals under the plan must be limited to $8,500 (in 2001) or $33^{1}/_{3}$ percent of the participant's includible compensation. The $8,500 limit is increased to $11,000 in 2002 and is increased in $1,000 increments thereafter through 2006. For individuals who are participants in more than one plan, this maximum deferral limit is coordinated with other plans, including 403(b) plans. As a result, executives in not-for-profit organizations are severely limited in their ability to make meaningful deferrals to eligible 457 plans. For-profit employers are usually able to provide their employees with more lucrative deferred compensation opportunities.

Tax Implications of Traditional Forms of Nonqualified Compensation

Whether or not a plan is "eligible" has significant tax consequences. In the case of an eligible 457 plan, amounts deferred are taxable to the participant when paid or otherwise made available. The treatment of eligible 457 plans is similar to the tax treatment of deferred compensation plans maintained by taxable employers. In the case of an ineligible plan (i.e., a plan that does not meet the requirements of an eligible plan), the deferred amounts are taxable in the first year in which there is no substantial risk of forfeiture of the rights to the compensation (generally when they become vested and regardless of whether the amounts are actually distributed).

Under Section 457(f), the rights of a person to compensation are subject to a *substantial risk of forfeiture*, if in order to receive the compensation, the person must promise to perform "substantial" services in the future. This definition goes further than the typical substantial risk of forfeiture definition for for-profit employers. For taxable employers, the fact that benefits are subject to the risk of loss to creditors is sufficient, and additional services are typically not required. However, under Section 457, additional services are required and the risk of loss to creditors alone is insufficient to defer taxation. As a result, participants in an ineligible 457 plan have a more limited deferral period than under a for-profit deferred compensation arrangement, and they can incur a tax liability prior to the actual receipt of their deferred account balance.

Advantages and Disadvantages of Cash-Based Deferred Compensation

The primary advantages and disadvantages of cash-based deferred compensation arrangements (either eligible or ineligible, as noted) include the following.

Advantages

- Significant deferral period for eligible Section 457 plans.
- Flexibility with regard to deferral amounts. (Ineligible plans enable highly compensated employees to make up for benefits lost due to qualified plan limits.)
- Linkage to results. (Plans can be structured with a select group of participants and can provide additional benefits based on service or the achievement of performance goals.)
- A chance of strong returns. (Generally, assets can be invested in competitive investments.)
- Relatively low cost. (These plans avoid commissions and fees associated with insurance-based products, and they have lower administrative and compliance costs compared to qualified plans.)

Disadvantages

- Risk of forfeiture and termination. (In a nonqualified plan, assets are subject to claims of the employer's creditors in the event of bankruptcy. That is, assets under these plans are not set aside in trusts and protected under the Employee Retirement Income Security Act (ERISA). A participant in a nonqualified plan is also not protected by ERISA rules regarding plan termination unless protected through mechanisms such as a rabbi trust.

- Limited employee participation. (By design, to avoid coverage by ERISA, these plans are limited to a select group of management.)
- No corporate tax deduction for nonqualified plans until the employee recognizes income.
- Taxability. (Income from amounts set aside to informally fund a plan for a taxable company is currently taxable, unless the investments are tax-sheltered.)
- Securities law and other legal considerations for certain plans.

One variation of the cash-based deferred compensation approach is to fund the benefit obligation with life insurance. This strategy, along with other common forms of insurance-based products, is discussed in the section below.

INSURANCE-BASED COMPENSATION ARRANGEMENTS

Life insurance coverage generally provides an assurance that, if accidents occur or disaster strikes, the insurance proceeds will be able to meet certain financial obligations. However, there is more to insurance than protection. For example, permanent life insurance can be a powerful tool for accumulating wealth on a tax-deferred basis, or for transferring wealth to heirs at a low-tax cost.

Many tax-exempt entities use permanent life insurance as a tool to create wealth for their executives. The cash value produced by permanent insurance policies accumulates tax-deferred wealth during the executive's lifetime, and, because of the tax characteristics of life insurance, can supplement the executive's retirement through policy cash withdrawals or policy loans. However, executives must be cautious in this regard—under certain circumstances, withdrawals or loans from the policy's cash values can cause the policy to lapse (terminate) in the future.

For most insurance contracts, a withdrawal of cash value is treated first as a return of principal (generally based on total premiums paid), so no taxable income is recognized until the total withdrawals from the policy exceed total premiums paid. Once this limit is reached, policy loans are taken out without recognizing any income, and the policy loans are repaid from the policy death benefit. Furthermore, life insurance death benefits are generally not subject to income tax. As such, they can be a powerful way for the executive's beneficiaries to accumulate capital.

This portion of the chapter examines several ways life insurance is structured in tax-exempt organizations to increase wealth. We focus on how life insurance allows the executive to access the policy's cash value in a tax-advantaged manner through policy withdrawals or policy loans. We also outline the income tax implications, advantages, and disadvantages of each benefit structure from the executive's perspective. Furthermore, we discuss the risk associated with using a strategy of policy withdrawals and policy loans to supplement executive retirement income. The more common executive benefit designs financed with life insurance include:

- Section 162 executive bonus plans,
- Split-dollar arrangements, and
- Ineligible Section 457 plans funded with life insurance.

Section 162 Bonus Plans

A Section 162 bonus plan, named after IRC Section 162 governing certain aspects of executive compensation, is simply an agreement between the employer and executive that requires the employer to award "bonus" compensation to the executive in an amount sufficient to pay life insurance premiums. (Of course, since this payment is promised in advance, the payment technically may not always be a true "bonus" in the usual performance-related sense, but this is the standard nomenclature for these plans.) The executive is the policy owner and has the right to all policy benefits, including the right to designate the policy beneficiary. The corporation has no interest in the policy.

In practice, the employer pays the premiums directly to the insurance carrier. As such, the bonus to the executive is in the form of those premium payments.

Typically, cash value policies (whole life or universal life) are used with this type of plan. Ideally, the policy is designed so that a limited number of future premiums will support the policy through retirement. The trend is to utilize variable universal life type policies because the cash value component of the life insurance can be allocated among various accounts similar to mutual funds. Since policy cash values build up tax free, these plans have similarities to Section 403(b) plans without the contribution limitations.

Section 162 can have favorable tax implications for the executive. The executive is the policy owner and the employer makes premium payments on the executive's behalf. As such, the executive recognizes taxable income equal to the amount of the premium paid. In cases where the employer "grosses up" the bonus to compensate for withholding taxes (that is, pays the employee an additional amount equal to the taxes withheld), the executive will be required to report both the premium and the gross-up amount as compensation income.

Other income tax implications Section 162 bonus plans:

- Death benefits received by the executive's designated beneficiary are not subject to income tax.
- Withdrawals of cash value are generally tax-free up to the executive's investment in the contract (usually total premiums deposited in the contract by the employer).[1]
- After the executive's total investment in the contract is withdrawn, further cash advances may be taken out in the form of tax-free policy loans. (Policy loan risk is discussed below.) Generally, there are no contributions or penalties for early withdrawal.[2]

Primary advantages and disadvantages of Section 162 bonus plans:

Advantages

- Administrative simplicity.
- Selectivity of participating executives.
- Individual design of plan benefit terms and conditions.
- Minimal ERISA and other Department of Labor reporting requirements.
- Insulation from claims of the employer's creditors.
- Insurance value for disability. (Under certain designs the insurance company will pay all premiums in the event the employee becomes permanently and totally disabled.)
- Liquidity. (The executive has the ability to access policy cash values via policy withdrawals or policy loans on a tax-free basis.)
- Portability. (The life insurance policy remains with the employee even if he/she changes employers.)

Disadvantages

- Lack of liquidity. (The employer cannot access policy cash values.)
- Performance risk. (The executive must accept all policy performance risks.)
- Dependence on executive's insurability. (Executive must have a certain level of insurability based on actuarial tables for age, health, etc.)

Split-Dollar Arrangements

Split-dollar arrangements are basically ways to buy life insurance. The term "split-dollar" encompasses a wide variety of plans where the employer and employee split the premium payment obligation and benefits of a life insurance contract. Death proceeds received by the employer/executive beneficiaries during the split-dollar arrangement—or after it terminates—are income tax free.

The split-dollar arrangement is not a separate type of life insurance. Rather, it is, as mentioned, a purchase arrangement. Although there are many variations of split-dollar, the most common methods of split-dollar are collateral assignment, endorsement, and reverse.

Collateral Assignment Split-Dollar Arrangements

The most common form of split-dollar is the *collateral assignment* method. Under this form of split-dollar, the employer normally pays all or most of the premium. In turn, the employer receives a share of the policy rights and benefits equal to the premium dollars it has advanced. The executive normally pays any premium due in excess of what the employer has paid and receives the lion's share of the death benefit—as well as interest in the policy's cash value in excess of the employer's interest. The portion paid, if any, by the executive is equal to the value of the economic benefit (VEB) that is derived from the insurance carrier's one-year term rate (OYT).

Under this method, when the split-dollar arrangement terminates (whether at the executive's death or during the executive's lifetime), the employer is reimbursed, without interest, through the policy's death benefit or cash surrender value. From the employer's perspective, the cost of the arrangement is the lost time value of money on the cumulative premiums paid. After the split-dollar arrangement is terminated and the employer is reimbursed, the executive has all rights to the remaining policy values. The executive may access policy cash values through policy withdrawals and/or policy loans to supplement retirement income.

Generally, the economics of collateral assignment split-dollar arrangements work best if the policy is designed with higher than normal premium payments during the first 10 policy years and the arrangement remains in force for at least 15 policy years. When properly designed, this allows the policy to accumulate sufficient cash value to reimburse the employer, provide for the executive retirement withdrawals and loans, and pay the costs of the life insurance product including commissions, mortality costs, and maintenance expenses.

Life insurance policy funding is normally based on certain assumptions regarding future policy performance. If the policy underperforms those assumptions, the premium funding design may not meet the policy's cashflow needs and could cause the policy to terminate without value, creating extremely unfavorable income tax results for the executive. Thus, split-dollar plans should be monitored annually to determine whether the growth of the policy's cash value is on track to meet its future demands. Because of the various tax risks associated with split-dollar arrangements, organizations should not implement these arrangements without the assistance of a tax advisor who understands them.

Some collateral assignment split-dollar arrangements are designed in tandem with special deferred compensation agreements geared to the arrangements. Such an agreement provides that if the executive meets certain age or service requirements, the executive will receive a deferred compensation benefit equal to the cumulative premiums paid by the employer under the split-dollar arrangement. Thus, the employer "funds" the deferred compensation plan through the return of premium obtained under the split-dollar arrangement.

Endorsement Split-Dollar Arrangements

The *endorsement* split-dollar method funds premiums the same way the collateral assignment does, but in this method, the employer owns the policy. Typically, the employer's death benefit is defined as the greater of the return of cumulative premiums or the policy's cash value. No cash value equity accrues to the executive. When the split-dollar arrangement terminates, the employer retains the policy.

Generally, employers use this form of split-dollar to provide an executive "death benefits only" plan while the executive maintains his/her employment. This form of split-dollar is also an informal way to fund the executive's retirement benefits. As policy owner, the employer accesses the policy's cash values through policy surrender, withdrawals, or loans to help fund the retirement benefit obligation.

Reverse Split-Dollar Arrangements

The *reverse* split-dollar form is similar to endorsement split-dollar, but with the parties reversed. The executive is the policy owner, has full rights to the policy's cash value, and pays the lion's share of the premium. The employer is the beneficiary of the death benefit in excess of the policy's cash value and pays the VEB based on the government's rates (now determined by Notice 2001-10, as explained below), rather than the insurance carrier's OYT rate. At termination, the executive takes over the entire policy. In practice, the employer usually pays the entire premium and treats the portion of the premium paid on behalf of the executive as compensation income.

Reverse split-dollar is sometimes used as a method of funding "key person" life insurance for a key employee. While the arrangement is in force, the employer's death benefit equals the excess of the total death benefit over the policy's cash value. This method of split-dollar is also used to provide a source of retirement income to the executive. The executive has full access to the policy's cash value, with no need to reimburse the employer when the split-dollar arrangement terminates. This provides the executive the unlimited right to access policy cash values through policy withdrawals or policy loans.

Tax Implications While Split-Dollar Arrangement is in Force

The taxation of collateral assignment and endorsement split-dollar arrangements depends, in part, on how the premium payments are arranged. If the employer pays the entire premium, the executive is required to report as imputed income the VEB under the split-dollar arrangement. The imputed income is offset to the extent of the executive's premium contributions. The VEB is based on annually increasing OYT insurance rates and thus, increases as the executive ages. The rates increase substantially when an executive reaches his/her mid-seventies, which is the primary reason why split-dollar arrangements should have a planned termination.

In addition to the taxability of the arrangement's economic benefit, executive taxation can arise if the policy pays policy dividends. Most practitioners believe, however, that this income can be avoided by including certain provisions under a properly drafted split-dollar agreement.

Under a reverse split-dollar arrangement, the employer has an interest in the policy's death benefit. As such, the employer is required to pay the cost (value) of the economic benefit (VEB) under the arrangement. The executive may pay the balance of the premium, but is not required to do so. If the employer pays the executive's portion of the premium, the executive must recognize this payment as compensation income.

Tax Implications when the Split-Dollar Agreement Terminates

Split-dollar agreements have special implications after termination. Collateral assignment plans may have either a *rollout* or a *release*.

- In the rollout approach to termination of a collateral assignment split-dollar plan, the split-dollar terminates when the employer is reimbursed. As previously indicated, the executive owns the policy under a collateral assignment split-dollar arrangement. Typically, the reimbursement is provided by partial policy surrenders or withdrawals. The executive has unlimited rights to the policy immediately after the corporation is reimbursed. Although most of the cash value is derived from premiums paid by the corporation, the executive should not be subject to a taxable event.

- In the release approach to termination of a collateral assignment split-dollar plan, the initial arrangement is structured with a release of the premium reimbursement obligation. Under this approach, the corporation cancels the executive's premium reimbursement obligation. The release is generally conditioned on meeting some type of age or service requirement. The executive recognizes income equal to the amount of premiums released when the condition to receiving the release is met. Income taxes on the income recognized by the executive are generally funded by policy withdrawals.

Endorsement split dollar arrangements terminate in a different way. Recall that under endorsement split-dollar method, the employer is the policy owner. When the arrangement terminates, the executive has no rights to the policy; all rights belong to the employer. As a result, the executive experiences no tax effect when the split-dollar arrangement terminates. In some cases, the life insurance policy is transferred out to the executive immediately after the endorsement split-dollar arrangement terminates. Under these circumstances, the executive recognizes taxable income equal to policy's cash value on the date of transfer.

The tax treatment for reverse split-dollar is similar to that discussed under the endorsement method above, only the parties are reversed. When the arrangement terminates, the employer gives up its rights to the policy's death benefit. Immediately after this occurs, all policy rights belong to the employee. The executive does not recognize a taxable event when the corporation releases its death benefit rights.

Income Tax Risk of Split-Dollar Plans

Split-dollar arrangements are not free from tax risk. The taxation of split-dollar life insurance arrangements is controlled by a small number of revenue rulings published by the Internal Revenue Service. There are several ways to interpret these rulings, and each interpretation implies a unique set of tax risks, advantages, and disadvantages.

For example, as this book went to press, the IRS issued Notice 2001-10 that may dramatically change the way split-dollar is treated for income taxation purposes. While the Notice is unclear on many fronts, one certain result will be a change in the rates the government uses to measure the taxable VEB received by employees from the pure insurance protection provided by split-dollar plans. The Notice eliminates the use of the insurance carrier's one-year term rates used to value compensation (VEB) in collateral assignment and endorsement split-dollar situations. Instead, the Notice requires the term rates used under these arrangements to reflect the rates of policies that are frequently sold to standard risks. (Previously, the government required only that the term rate used for the VEB be a published rate available to standard risks.)

Another change was the replacement of the government's own PS 58 rates, first established by the Internal Revenue Service's Pension Service a half century ago. The Notice said that the IRS will no longer accept the PS 58 table rate, and has issued interim one-year term premium insurance rates (Table 2001) as a substitute for the outdated P S 58 rates. The Table 2001 rates are much lower than the PS 58 rates and, if applied under a reverse split-dollar arrangement, would substantially reduce the employer's premium.

The Notice also indicates that an employee may be required to report additional income to account for the employee's interest in the policy's cash value. Therefore, the Notice requires an employer to treat its premium payments as either interest-free loans, as an investment in the contract for the employer's own account, or as compensation to the employee. If the arrangement is treated as an interest-free loan, the employer's forgone interest on the "premium loans" will be treated as compensation income to the insured/employee. No further income is recognized by the insured/employee. If the arrangement is not treated as an interest-free loan, not only will the insured/employee recognize income equal the VEB, but, pending further IRS guidance, the policy's cash value growth in excess of premiums may also be deemed as compensation income.

It is expected that the life insurance industry will expend great efforts to have this Notice withdrawn or modified. Unfortunately, it is impossible to predict how this controversy will ultimately be settled.

Loan and Policy Performance Risk of Split-Dollar Plans

Another technique for wealth accumulation involves borrowing money on a life insurance policy. This is a risky strategy that should be pursued with care. Although policy loan and policy performance risk applies to any cash value life insurance policy (whole life, universal, or variable universal life), the risk is magnified with variable universal life insurance policies. These policies are more susceptible to volatility because the cash values are invested in sub-accounts (similar to mutual funds) and are generally subject to greater market risk.

Variable life insurance policies provide no guarantee of investment performance or minimum cash values. Policy cash values can decrease substantially due to unfavorable investment performance and may cause the policy to terminate prematurely. When policy loans are added into the equation, the accrued loan interest increases the stress on the policy's cash values. If the policy terminates during life with an outstanding loan balance, any gain on the policy becomes immediately taxable to the policy owner.

Advantages and Disadvantages of Split-Dollar Plans

Advantages

- Low cost retirement benefit to executive.
- Selectivity of participating executives.
- Low premium payment relative to the death benefit coverage for executive.
- Tax-free cash value withdrawals and loans for executive.
- Relatively low taxable income to executive.
- Tax-free death benefits to executive's heirs.
- A substantial risk of forfeiture on the policy benefits may not be required.
- Under collateral assignment and reverse split-dollar, the executive's equity in the policy's cash value is not subject to the claims of the employer's creditors.

Disadvantages

- Tax and policy performance risks.
- Compensation under the arrangement increases annually.
- Collateral assignment split-dollar plans generally need to be in force 15 years or longer.
- High annual cash flows are required under the collateral assignment split-dollar method to properly fund the policy. This disadvantage can be diminished if the arrangement is structured with a release. However, the release creates additional taxable income to the employee.
- Life insurance products contain mortality and other insurance company expenses.
- The plans are somewhat inflexible. When an executive's employment terminates unexpectedly, the policy may not provide much, if any, equity for the executive.

- The executive may be required to recognize taxable income if substantial policy withdrawals take place within the policy's first 15 policy years.
- Complexity of the arrangement compared to non-insurance based plans.
- Uncertainty of tax treatment given the recent notice.

INELIGIBLE SECTION 457 PLANS FUNDED WITH LIFE INSURANCE

As discussed in other sections of this chapter, IRC Section 457(f) exempts ineligible Section 457 plans from the annual deferral limitations imposed under Section 457. As a result, an employer can defer an unlimited amount of executive compensation, as long as the benefits are subject to a substantial risk of forfeiture. This means that if the executive terminates employment prior to retirement before fulfilling a length of service commitment, non-compete agreement, etc., the executive will forfeit the deferred compensation benefits.

An employer may purchase life insurance to indemnify the cost it incurs to fund the executive's deferred compensation benefit. Life insurance policies covering key executives also offset some of the organization's financial hardship that results when an executive dies unexpectedly. In many respects, the benefits to the employer resemble those provided under the endorsement split-dollar approach discussed above except the employer maintains all policy rights and death benefits.

To understand how ineligible Section 457 plans work, it is important to remember that two types of deferred compensation plans exist; salary continuation plans and salary reduction plans. The tax implications are the same for both plans. Where they differ is in how the benefit is funded. Under a salary continuation plan, the employer dollars usually fund the benefit, whereas with a salary reduction plan, executive deferrals fund the insurance. This distinction is relevant to the tax implications of ineligible Section 457 plans.

Tax Implications of Ineligible Section 457 Plans

In an ineligible Section 457 plan, since the employer is the policy owner, the policy itself does not create any tax implication to the executive. Instead, the executive's taxation is governed by the terms of the deferred compensation agreement. An executive participating in an ineligible Section 457 deferred compensation plan will not be taxed until the substantial risk of forfeiture on those benefits is released—because the executive fulfills the required service commitment. At that time the benefit is payable unconditionally. The tax results for the executive do not change when the employer uses life insurance to finance the deferred compensation benefit.

In a salary reduction plan, the executive should elect to reduce his/her salary in advance—that is, prior to the time the employee performs the services that are compensated by the salary. If the executive has already performed the services, the IRS will probably not recognize the amount of the salary reduction as a tax-free deferral under Section 457.

An ineligible Section 457 Plan beneficiary is taxed on the total amount of plan benefits in the year that the executive dies. This tax treatment results even if the employer uses policy death benefits to fund the plan benefit payment. Although the death benefit proceeds to the employer maintain their tax-free characteristics, these characteristics are lost when the proceeds are subsequently transferred to the executive's ineligible Section 457 Plan beneficiary.

Advantages and Disadvantages of Insurance-Funded Ineligible Section 457 Plans

There are advantages and disadvantages of ineligible Section 457 plans funded with life insurance.

Advantages

- Employer reimbursement for cost of deferred compensation benefits.
- A greater level of assurance (through a formal insurance contract compared with a mere contractual promise) that the benefit will be paid.
- Employer access to policy cash values for general business purposes.

Disadvantages

- High cost of annual premium payments if the participant pool is large.
- Vulnerability to claims of the employer's creditors.

MUTUAL FUND OPTION PLANS

A relatively recent alternative in the area of deferred compensation for tax-exempt employers involves the grant of an option to transfer property, such as shares in a mutual fund at a discounted strike price. The basic premise of such a program is that the tax treatment is governed by Section 83, which applies to all compensatory transfers of property, rather than by Section 457.[3] This enables the participant to benefit from long deferral periods, avoid the limitations of eligible Section 457 plans, and gain control over the timing and amount of income recognition. From the organization's perspective, such a plan provides the opportunity for a flexible and competitive compensation program.

Typically, the organization adopts an option plan for the benefit of a select group of key employees, and enters into separate option agreements with these individuals. These agreements provide the opportunity to purchase a certain quantity and type of financial product (e.g., shares in a mutual fund) at a specified price. The organization determines the exercise price of the option (generally at a discount of 50 to 75 percent), which can either remain fixed over the term of the option or can be adjusted to maintain the original discount. The ultimate value of the option depends on the appreciation in the underlying property.

As with other forms of stock options, the participant elects the time of exercise, tendering the exercise price in order to receive delivery of the underlying property (following the completion of any vesting period and prior to the expiration of the option). At the time of exercise, the participant can either hold the shares or immediately sell them. The option can contain features to encourage retention (e.g., vesting schedules) or the accomplishment of performance objectives (e.g., incentive-based awards). Because this benefit involves the purchase and sale of securities, organizations implementing such plans should consider the impact of federal and state securities laws.

While the mutual fund option plan can be applicable to for-profit companies, such a plan is subject to unfavorable financial statement accounting treatment and has been more widely used in the nonprofit community. For-profit companies adopting option plans will typically award options on the employer's own stock.

Nonprofit organizations implementing a mutual fund option plan need to assess the plan's implications for reasonable compensation in light of the proposed Intermediate Sanctions regulations (Internal Revenue Code Section 4958), private inurement, and private benefit implications. (For more information on these subjects, see Chapter 4.)

Tax Implications of Mutual Fund Option Plans

Mutual fund option plans are designed to be covered by IRC Section 83. The granting of the option is not itself a taxable event because the option does not have a value that is "readily ascertainable." The employee recognizes ordinary income at the date of exercise of the option in an amount equal to the excess of the fair market value (measured at the time of exercise) of the financial product over the exercise price. Any appreciation between the dates of exercise and sale is taxed at capital gains tax rates (either short-term or long-term depending on the holding period).

Advantages and Disadvantages of Mutual Fund Option Plans

Employers should weigh the advantages and disadvantages of option programs.

Advantages

- Employer flexibility with plan design (retention features, forfeiture restrictions, eligibility, deferral amounts, and performance-based awards).
- Employee control over timing of income recognition and access to vested assets.
- Applicability to both short-term and long-term deferrals.
- Lack of commissions and fees associated with insurance-based products.
- Mix of current and deferred compensation.

Disadvantages

- Lack of tax-free death benefit associated with insurance products.
- Potential for IRS or legislative challenge that may require the application of Section 457.

- Risk of low investment performance of underlying asset.
- Administrative burden associated with large option plans.
- Potential negative publicity associated with stock options (especially in a tax-exempt organization).

CONCLUSION

Healthcare organizations face considerable competition in their search for leadership talent. Compensation offers one way to compete for that talent through dollars. The most astute organizations, however, are not paying all those dollars today. Instead, they are offering their executives various forms of deferred compensation, including qualified and nonqualified plans, insurance-based products, and mutual fund option plans. In this way, the organizations achieve a balance between their executive's financial goals and their own business goals.

NOTES

1. All or a portion of any cash withdrawals received within the first 15 policy years may be subject to income tax under the forced-out gain provisions of IRC Section 7702(f)(7).

2. Policies that fail a "seven-pay test" under IRC Section 7702A become modified endowment contracts (MEC). Distributions (including cash value withdrawals, policy surrenders or policy loans) from MECs are treated as a distribution of policy earnings first and as a recovery of basis (i.e., investment in the contract) to the extent of the excess. A 10 percent penalty tax may also apply to the extent income is recognized on a MEC distribution if the distribution occurs prior to the policy owner's age 59$^{1}/_{2}$.

3. There are a number of exceptions to the coverage of deferred compensation arrangements under Section 457, including plans described in Sections 401(a), 402(b), 403, and 415(m).

CHAPTER 6

Executive Employment Contracts in Healthcare

Douglas M. Mancino

DURING THE PAST decade, employment contracts between healthcare organizations and their executives have become increasingly formal. Gone are the days of "handshake" employment deals consummated over a friendly dinner and memorialized in a three-paragraph confirming letter. A competitive marketplace for qualified executives, consolidation within the healthcare industry, a changing legal landscape (with a growing number of laws pertaining to age and sex discrimination and other issues), and an increasingly and appropriately "businesslike" environment have contributed to a change in the way healthcare systems and their current and prospective senior executives approach the negotiation and documentation of employment arrangements.

The overall marketplace for qualified healthcare executives has changed as well. A generation ago, it was not unusual for an individual, typically male, to accept an offer of employment after the completion of his administrative residency at a hospital and, over a few years, work his way to one of the senior or top leadership positions at the same hospital. There, the individual typically would have had a relatively stable career path and remained with the hospital until his retirement. Today, that career path of hospital executives of old seems as antiquated as a Model T Ford. Rather, the typical career path of a talented male or female healthcare executive is punctuated by frequent career- or family-driven moves, and the "half-life" of healthcare CEOs is frequently measured in a number of years that can be counted on one hand.

Finally, as in many areas of business, decisions of healthcare systems and their executives with respect to executive compensation are affected by, and sometimes based entirely on, tax-planning considerations and developments. Not-for-profit tax-exempt healthcare systems in particular must take into consideration myriad tax issues, including Section 4958 of the Internal Revenue Code (IRC), which sets requirements for avoiding "intermediate sanctions" that can be levied for unreasonable compensation, and IRC Section 457, which places significant constraints on certain unfunded deferred compensation arrangements available to executives of not-for-profit healthcare systems. (For more information on these topics, see Chapter 4, which covers the new temporary regulations on intermediate sanctions, and Chapter 5 on deferred compensation.)

This chapter explores the issues and considerations that make up the development of an employment relationship between a healthcare organization and its senior executives. Some of the matters discussed in this chapter should be a part of any employment relationship between a healthcare system and its senior executives, particularly the chief executive officer (CEO), while others should be up to the discretion of the executive and the institution.

SHOULD THE EMPLOYMENT CONTRACT BE IN WRITING?

One of the most basic decisions that a healthcare institution must make is the decision whether to put the employment contract with the CEO or other senior executives in writing.

As a matter of basic employment law, an employment contract does not have to be in writing to be enforceable. In many jurisdictions, a verbal agreement and "handshake" may be considered an acceptable contract. Furthermore, most employment relationships generate some "written" proof of a contractual relationship, even if the individual and the health system do not sign a definitive employment contract. The employee may receive employee policies and handbooks, for example. Also, the employee may benefit from a qualified retirement plan that extends to all health system employees, from the CEO to the entry-level employee, irrespective of whether the individual is a full or part-time employee.

Reliance on a verbal agreement or ancillary documents, while possible, is unwise. There are important reasons for considering the use of written employment contracts for the CEO of the health system, as well as for the other senior members of the management team, such as the chief operating officer, chief financial officer, and human resources director.

The American College of Healthcare Executive states, in its classic publication *Contracts for Healthcare Executives,* that "executive employment contracts are a needed mechanism to ensure organizations are led and managed by those unafraid to take bold initiatives."[1]

Our own experience in practicing the law of contracts in the healthcare arena confirms this conclusion for three main reasons (discussed in more detail later on in this chapter):

1. Both the healthcare organization and the senior executive are typically entering into the employment relationship with the expectation that the health system will enjoy the services of the senior executive for a period of years, and the senior executive will have the commitment from the organization to remain in its employ for a period of years, subject to the fulfillment of his or her executive responsibilities. It would be highly unusual for persons seeking senior executive positions to expect to be treated as "at-will" hires.

2. A written agreement can help the executive and the healthcare organization avoid any ambiguity about the key terms

of the employment relationship, such as compensation, duration of employment, and duties and responsibilities. The written employment contract can also memorialize important agreements about post-employment issues, such as an agreement not to compete, an agreement to preserve the confidentiality of trade secrets, and an agreement not to solicit the health system's employees or interfere with outside contractual relationships, such as contracts with managed care organizations. This chapter will discuss all these points in greater detail.

3. A written agreement, under certain circumstances, can clarify the timing of an agreement with respect to tax regulations. For example, it can prevent some parts of the executive's compensation from being considered as part of a compensation total subject to intermediate sanctions regulations with regard to "excessive compensation" or "excess benefits," as discussed further below.

COMPENSATION ELEMENTS TYPICALLY COVERED IN A WRITTEN CONTRACT

A well-drafted employment contract between a health system and its CEO or other senior executives will address several major compensation components, many of which will actually be addressed in separate written agreements. These separate agreements may be drafted specifically for the organization's relationship with a particular employee, or they may apply to all employees in general. The overall legal structure of the compensation contract itself will be discussed later in this chapter. In this section, we will examine the main points to be covered— or at least referenced—in a contract.

As discussed in Chapter 2, there are four main elements of compensation: cash compensation, benefits, equity compensation, and perquisites. The employment contract may cover some or all of these areas.

Cash Compensation

An executive employment contract may specify the amount of pay to be received in base salary, incentive compensation, and bonuses (all typically paid in cash). As discussed in Chapter 2, these elements interact with other pay elements as part of total compensation.

Benefits

One useful purpose of a written contract is to memorialize agreements concerning benefits, especially deferred compensation, severance pay, and change-of-control plans.

Deferred compensation

The qualified retirement plans of most not-for-profit health systems are typically geared toward providing retirement benefits to rank and file employees, not to executive-level employees—particularly the most senior executives. As a consequence, a critical element of any competitive employment relationship will be the deferred compensation arrangements put in place for the benefit of the CEO and, quite frequently, the senior management team of a health system.

One typical element of the deferred compensation/retirement package for senior-level executives is the IRC Section 403(b) tax-sheltered annuity program that is generally available to all health-care organization employees. These programs are offered and administered by insurance companies, and typically the insurers will provide the written documentation. Nonetheless, contracts between healthcare organizations and their senior executives often do cover this area. The issue of contribution allocation—how much the employer will contribute versus how much the executive will contribute—will typically be addressed in writing as part of the regular employment arrangement.

Some organizations find it desirable to offer their senior executives additional deferred compensation beyond these annuity programs. Indeed, the current competitive environment for senior healthcare executives often demands the adoption of some form of additional deferred compensation arrangement for the chief executive officer, at a minimum, and possibly other senior-level members of the management team as well.

These deferred compensation arrangements are typically unfunded pension plans, or pension plans that are funded by transferring monies to a separate trust, known as a "rabbi trust." These plans, whether unfunded or funded, are typically designed to meet the requirements of IRC Section 457, and thus to include a "substantial risk of forfeiture." That is, the amounts remain subject to the claims of creditors of the health system and thus are subject to the solvency and other risks of the health system. Indeed, it is an unfortunate fact of life today that hospitals and health systems can go into bankruptcy and become insolvent and go out of business. Consequently, the healthcare organization may put in place for one or more of its senior executives an after-tax retirement benefit program that is *not* accessible by the creditors of the organization.

Severance pay

Another common benefit to frequently appear in contracts between healthcare organizations and their senior executives is a severance pay benefit. This benefit is particularly attractive to tax-exempt health systems and their employees because, if properly structured, it can qualify as a "bona fide" severance pay plan under Section 457, which contains an exception for such plans. Importantly, a bona fide severance pay plan cannot exceed the individual's highest W-2 compensation during the preceding two years, prior to his or her severance from employment. Also, importantly, a plan will not qualify as a severance pay plan if it really kicks in at retirement, according to the IRS.

A severance benefit or a separate severance plan should be in writing to avoid ambiguity concerning the terms of its availability, the individuals to which it is applicable, and other factors.

Change-of-control plans

Yet another feature in executive employment contracts is a clause guaranteeing continued compensation in a change-of-control. This clause might be considered discretionary, especially among not-for-profits, which rarely include it in employment contracts. Nonetheless, it is important to recognize the existence of such clauses, and to consider their merits.

As mentioned at the outset of this chapter, consolidation in the healthcare industry has helped change the relationship between healthcare institutions and executives. For example, two common assumptions have been shattered: first, the assumption that the freestanding hospital for which the individual serves as an executive would always remain freestanding and independent; and second, the assumption that a long-standing not-for-profit hospital (or other healthcare institution) would never consider selling out to an investor-owned or other for-profit company.

For these reasons, many healthcare systems (including not-for-profits) have adopted "change-of-control" or similar plans that are expressly intended to provide compensation, health and welfare, retirement, and other benefits to senior-level executives in the event that the board of directors of the healthcare system decides to sell or otherwise dispose of control (e.g., through a membership transfer) to another not-for-profit or taxable hospital or healthcare system.

Change-of-control plans benefit healthcare organizations and executives alike because, at least conceptually, they relieve the senior executive or executives from the concern that they may lose their employment. This reduces the risk that they will simply leave the organization prematurely for a more secure organization, and it reduces the risk that the employee will attempt, overtly or, typically, subtly, to subvert the change-of-control plans.

Signing and retention bonuses

If these bonuses are offered, they may be described in the contract. Defining the circumstances under which these bonuses will and will not be payable is important.

KEY PARTS OF A WRITTEN EMPLOYMENT CONTRACT

There is no "cookie-cutter" form of employment contract that will meet the needs of every health system with respect to every senior executive. While it may be useful to start with an employment contract form, the organization must realize that each employment arrangement is unique. (Any employer that fails to recognize this will get a prompt reminder of this from the recruited executive!)

The following paragraphs discuss a number of items, most of which will be found in any well drafted written employment contract. Some of them, however, are discretionary.

Duties and Responsibilities

Every employment contract should contain one or more paragraphs that describe the individual's duties and responsibilities. Obviously, the obligation on the part of the health system to compensate and provide other benefits to the employee is contingent upon his or her performance of his or her duties and responsibilities to the organization. While the employment contract may describe the individual's position as "president," "vice president," or "chief financial officer," usually those descriptions of positions are not adequate.

At a minimum, the contract should include a brief position description that is consistent with (and possibly based on) the corporate bylaws of the health system. In most instances, the position should be described in greater detail, particularly since other elements of the compensation plan, such as bonuses, may be contingent upon fulfillment of the responsibilities of the position. In addition, many employees will want to see their reporting relationship documented in the employment contract. For example, a newly hired vice president and general counsel will, in all likelihood, want to know whether he or she is reporting directly to the CEO, to the COO, or to the CFO. These reporting relationship issues typically become more important and heavily negotiated when an individual is being hired by a health system with multiple operating units.

Term, Termination, and Renewals

The written employment agreement should be clear about the initial term of the agreement, as well as renewal periods. From a legal point of view, no restrictions exist on the duration of the initial or renewal terms of an employment agreement. Organizations and executives should bear in mind, however, that the initial and renewal terms, particularly if renewals occur automatically, will be factors in the overall determination of whether compensation paid or payable to an executive is reasonable. While a 5-year initial term with one 5-year renewal may overall be reasonable, a 15- or 20-year initial term may be considered, per se, unreasonable. This is especially true if the health system may not terminate it without cause.

In addition, it is critical for the health system and the employee to agree upon appropriate grounds for termination of the employment agreement prior to the expiration of its term or renewals. Normally, every employment agreement will be terminable for cause, and it is useful to decide in advance what constitutes cause and what does not. (The author has seen employment contracts between a health system and its CEO that were terminable only if the executive becomes something just short of a serial killer. Conversely, the author has seen contracts that defined cause so broadly that even a saint would have trouble maintaining a position.) While unusual, these contracts can and do happen unless the organization and the executive adopt a balanced approach.

Such an approach generally involves a definition of "just cause" that relates to nonperformance or inadequate performance by the executive of his or her duties with respect to the organization, violations of law (particularly healthcare laws applicable to the organization), and engagement in acts of moral turpitude that would, in some fashion, affect the ability of the individual to carry out his or her responsibilities to the organization.

The contract's treatment of term, termination, and renewal should be drafted with due attention to tax law. In particular, drafters should bear in mind the "initial contract" exception in the temporary intermediate sanctions rules under IRC Section 4958. This section sets forth certain conditions under which a not-for-profit executive might be deemed to receive "excessive compensation" or "excess benefits" that would not be consistent with the tax-exempt status of the not-for-profit.

As detailed in Chapter 4, one of the key questions addressed in these temporary regulations is the status of individuals as "qualified" or "disqualified" with respect to the tax-exempt healthcare organization. If an individual is considered "disqualified," his or her relationship with the healthcare system becomes subject to the intermediate sanctions rules and potential penalties. The "initial contract" exception in the temporary regulations is applicable to written agreements put in place between a health organization and its senior executives prior to the time they undertake their responsibilities with the organization.

Under these temporary regulations, the initial contract will not be subject to intermediate sanctions with respect to matters such as compensation and benefits addressed in the written contract, unless and until the contract is terminable by the health system without cause or penalty.

The exception applies to employment as well as other forms of contracts that are in writing between a tax-exempt organization and its senior executive-level employees. However, this initial contract exception extends only until the tax-exempt employer has the ability to terminate the employment agreement without penalty. Thus, for example, if a 5-year employment contract is terminable after 3 years upon giving 90 days written notice without penalty, the maximum period to which the initial contract exception would apply in this example would be 3 years plus 90 days, because after the giving of 90-days notice at the end of the 3-year period, the not-for-profit health system could (even if it chose not to) terminate the employment agreement without penalty.

This initial contract exception applies to contingent compensation arrangements, such as bonuses, that are payable to the executive pursuant to a formula. Importantly, however, it does not apply to bonus arrangements that are discretionary.

Compensation

For reasons that should be obvious, the compensation provisions of an employment agreement are typically the provisions that receive the most attention before, during, and at the end of an employment relationship.

Compensation provisions in an employment agreement will include fixed or base compensation, contingent compensation, health and welfare benefits, retirement benefits, and a number of other types of compensation, depending upon the circumstances.

For example, provisions may promise to make up lost pay or benefits, or to provide other benefits, such as reimbursement of moving expenses, tax reimbursement, financial and estate-planning advice, and the like.

All compensation, regardless of form, will be considered in determining the overall reasonableness of compensation. Both organizations and their executives will want to make sure that neither the level of pay nor the nature of pay arrangements jeopardize the continued tax-exempt status of the not-for-profit healthcare system, or subjects the executive to intermediate sanctions under IRC Section 5498.

A well-crafted contract will do what it can to minimize the risk of intermediate sanctions. One way is to avoid including any clauses that will prevent the above-mentioned "initial contract" exception to the excessive compensation and excess benefit transactions. For example, it might include base compensation that is subject to annual raises tied to increases in the cost of living, because this will not jeopardize the initial contract exception availability. On the other hand, it would not offer base compensation increases that are discretionary, since such a provision will jeopardize the availability of the initial contract exception. Similarly, contingent compensation arrangements that use a pre-agreed formula will not jeopardize the availability of the initial contract exception, but contingent compensation arrangements that are discretionary will jeopardize the availability of that exception.

The provisions of a written employment contract are probably the most critical elements focused on during the negotiation of an initial employment agreement or the renegotiation of an existing employment agreement. However, there are three additional provisions that deserve more attention than they typically receive during the negotiation or renegotiation stages. These provisions may seem innocuous, but they can actually do harm if they are not well crafted, as explained below.

Choice of Law

Some contracts contain provisions specifying which law will prevail in the event of dispute. These "choice-of-law" provisions are rare in contracts involving a single, independent healthcare institution negotiating or renegotiating an employment agreement with a resident of the state in which the hospital is located. However, if a healthcare system conducts business across state lines, as many do, or if the system is recruiting an executive from out of state, the parties should reach a clear agreement on the choice of which law will be used to interpret the agreement, other than in those instances where federal law applies. The reason for this is simple. The laws of the states are not uniform, and some states may have been more aggressive in their efforts to protect individuals against age discrimination, sex discrimination, or other forms of discrimination, such as discrimination based on race or sexual preference. As a consequence, the choice of the state laws to which the employment agreement should be subject will typically be made based on the location in which the principal place of business of the employer is located.

Arbitration/Mediation

A closely related topic is the use of recognized alternate forms of dispute resolution. Instead of going to court, some parties to disputes are using experts in arbitration and mediation. To encourage such an alternative, those involved in drafting employment contracts should consider including a provision that states that arbitration and/or mediation will be required for all disputes, and naming the entity that will be controlling the arbitration or mediation.

Legal Costs

Another discretionary provision sometimes found in employment agreements is a provision that will award legal costs to the employee if he or she is successful in challenging his or her termination. Absent an express provision for reimbursement of legal fees and of other costs, or an express statutory requirement in a federal, state, or local law or ordinance, an individual would not normally be entitled to reimbursement of legal fees or costs to challenge a termination or other contractual dispute.

PARTING OF THE WAYS: POST-EMPLOYMENT PROVISIONS

The demand for qualified individuals to fill senior executive positions in health systems continues to be highly competitive. This fact, combined with realities that individuals may have many careers well beyond age 65, compel the not-for-profit health system to address openly and clearly the issues that will govern the relationship with the executive after he or she leaves the organization, voluntarily or otherwise. Many of the issues discussed below may be governed by other legal arenas, such as federal laws regarding discrimination, state laws regarding employment, or common law regarding wrongdoing ("tort" law) or a breach of contract. Nonetheless, employment contracts should address some or all of these matters.

Covenants Not to Compete

A covenant not to compete is an agreement by the individual not to engage in activities as an employee, as a shareholder, as a partner, as an independent contractor, or in any other capacity that will be competitive with the business or businesses of the health systems. As can be seen from the very ambiguity of the preceding sentence, the issues pertaining to covenants not to compete are quite important.

First, and possibly of most critical importance, is the need to be clear in defining what types of businesses the health system would consider competitive. Is it the operation of a hospital? Is it the operation of a clinical laboratory?

Second, a covenant not to compete will typically be governed by temporal as well as geographic limitations. A temporal limitation is typically one that says that the employee may not compete with the former employee for a period of one or two years after he or she has his or her employment terminated for any reason. A geographic limitation may take a wide range of forms, depending upon the definition of what constitutes competition. For example, the individual may be precluded from accepting employment by another hospital or health facility that is located within five miles of the hospital or health facility at which the person had previously served as an executive. Alternatively, the person may be precluded from accepting employment or otherwise providing services to any healthcare provider located in the same county of the state in which the individual was employed. Indeed, there may be situations in which a statewide or even national geographic limitation may be appropriate.

Healthcare organizations must be cautious here, however, because the laws and courts of most states tend to be employee-oriented. In some cases, state laws may even preclude the use of covenants not to compete in an employment contract. In any event, even in those states where such covenants are permitted by statute or under common law, organization should prepare to face considerable scrutiny on the temporal, geographic, and activity limitations expressed in these covenants.

Trade Secrets and Confidential Information

Senior executives of healthcare organizations come in contact with trade secrets and other confidential information of the hospital or health system as part of the conduct of their routine executive activities. Generally, the laws of most, if not all, states will have statutory or common law doctrines that can be invoked to prevent a former hospital executive from using trade secrets or other confidential information for his or her own benefit, or for the benefit of a new employer or partner.

Notwithstanding the existence of state statutes or common law doctrines, healthcare systems should try to prevent and punish inappropriate use of trade secrets and confidential information for personal or other benefit. Organizations can do this in employment contracts, personnel handbooks, and other appropriate locations. Moreover, when a written employment contract with a senior healthcare executive addresses exploitation or misappropriation of "trade secrets" and "confidential information," it is important to define these terms. Also, it is a good practice to define the legal remedies available to the organization in the event that an employee does make inappropriate use of the company's intellectual property.

Non-Solicitation

Employment contracts with senior executive-level employees should also prohibit the employee from soliciting the healthcare system's employees or customers (e.g., managed care organizations) after termination of his or her employment with the system.

CONCLUSION

The era of handshake employment deals in the healthcare industry ended, for most organizations, many, many years ago. In its place, the marketplace and changing business environment compel the devotion of more time, effort, and resources to the design and structure of employment agreements between health systems and their senior executives.

In this chapter, we have attempted to identify and discuss critical issues that should be part of any employment contract negotiations or discussions. To assist the reader, we have included a relatively "standard" form of employment contract as Appendix 6A. We also include two appendices related to change of control: Appendix 6B1 addresses the peculiar structural and other requirements found in the not-for-profit health system context; and Appendix 6B2, a contract relating change-of-control. As with any "form" or "standard" agreement, those terms should be taken with a grain of salt. When a healthcare institution and an executive make the commitment to form a relationship, they should rely on more than a handshake. Instead, they should craft an agreement that reflects and protects the full potential of their relationship, for the good of both parties.

NOTE

1. *Contracts for Healthcare Executives, Fourth Edition* (ACHE 2002), discusses the growing prevalence of employment contracts for healthcare CEOs and the trends fueling this growth. The higher level of risk involved in the operations and oversight of hospitals and healthcare organizations has made employment contracts more attractive to both executives and employers. Employment agreements can offer protections that enable executives to take prudent risks in making controversial but necessary changes. Likewise, the protections help employers attract and retain effective executives. New challenges arising since publication of the third edition include changes in control due to mergers and

acquisitions, growth in use of incentive compensation, and new perspectives on severance arrangements. Model contracts and letters of agreements in the appendices have been updated to reflect these challenges.

Employment Agreement

This Employment Agreement (this "Agreement") is effective as of _____, 200_ (the "Effective Date"), by and between New Era Health System, a California corporation ("Employer"), and _____, a resident of _____, _____, California ("Employee"), under the following terms and conditions:

WHEREAS, Employer and Employee desire to enter into this Agreement pursuant to which Employee will render services to Employer on the terms and conditions set forth herein.

NOW THEREFORE, in consideration of the mutual promises, covenants and agreements set forth below, it is hereby agreed as follows:

1.   <u>Employment</u>. Employer hereby employs Employee as _____ of Employer. Employee agrees to render such services to Employer as may be required by the above-referenced position, including but not limited to those duties set forth on Exhibit A, attached hereto, and such other duties incidental thereto as Employer or the Board of Directors or an executive officer of Employer may from time to time reasonably request Employee to assume. Employee agrees to serve Employer faithfully, diligently and to the best of his ability, and to faithfully adhere to, execute and fulfill all policies established by Employer.

2.   <u>Term of Employment</u>. Subject to the provisions of Sections 9 and 10 of this Agreement, Employee's employment under this Agreement shall be deemed to have commenced on the

Effective Date and continue for a period of one (1) year thereafter (the "Term"); provided, however, that Employer shall have the option, at its sole election, to extend this Agreement for successive one (1) year periods, by providing Employee written notice of such election not less than sixty (60) days prior to the end of the Term or any extensions thereof.

3. Compensation.

(a)   Base Salary. Employer shall pay Employee an annualized salary of _____ Dollars ($_____) (the "Base Salary"). The Base Salary will be paid by Employer to Employee in equal installments payable in accordance with the regular payroll policies of Employer in effect during the term of this Agreement, less applicable tax withholdings or other deductions required by law or authorized by Employee. The Base Salary may be increased, on an annual basis, but only in the sole discretion of the Board of Directors of Employer. The aforesaid reference to the Base Salary as being annualized or being increased on an annual basis is not intended and shall not be deemed as creating any term of employment under this Agreement other than as specifically set forth in Section 2, above.

(b)   Incentive Bonus. Within its sole discretion, Employer may pay Employee a performance bonus, which shall be paid, after evaluation by Employer, on the basis of a combination of objective and subjective criteria to be determined by Employer.

4. Working Hours.

(a)   Normal Working Hours. Employee will normally be expected to work a minimum of 37.5 hours per week. Normal working hours shall be from 9 a.m. to 5:30 p.m., Monday through Friday, with a one-hour lunch period to be taken between the hours of 12 p.m. and 2 p.m. Employer reserves the right to alter Employee's normal working hours in accordance with the need and requirements of the business and will notify Employee of any such change in the manner set forth in Section 21.

(b)   Additional Working Hours. Employee may be required to work outside of normal working hours if the requirements of the Employer's business so demands. Employee shall not be entitled to receive any additional remuneration for any work performed outside of normal working hours.

5.   Place of Employment. Employee's normal place of work will be at _____, CA _____. Employer reserves the right to change Employee's place of work to such location, within reasonable commuting distance of _____, as Employer may from time to time advise Employee. Employee may be required to travel throughout and outside the United States in the performance of his duties.

6.   Benefits. In addition to the compensation provided for in Section 3 above, Employer shall provide Employee with employment benefits of the type provided to employees of Employer generally during the Term, including but not limited to, eligibility for any vacation and sick leave benefits and participation in any health, life, disability insurance plans, and stock options whether now in effect or subsequently adopted, subject to Employer's right to amend, alter or terminate such Plans.

7.   Expenses. Employer shall pay all reasonable expenses properly incurred by Employee in furtherance of the business of the Employer, including traveling and entertainment expenses, and shall reimburse Employee monthly for all such expenses paid or incurred by Employee during the preceding month upon delivery of in appropriate expense report and receipts to Employer.

8.   Vacation. Subject to the adoption of a plan governing vacation benefits, vacation shall accrue to Employee at a rate of twenty (20) vacation days for each twelve (12) month period

from January 1 through December 31 (a Vacation Accrual Period) that Employee is employed by Employer or, if Employee has been employed for less than a complete Vacation Accrual Period, 1.6 vacation days shall accrue for each complete month of service within such Vacation Accrual Period. Vacation accrued but not taken by an Employee during any Vacation Accrual Period may not be carried forward to the following Vacation Accrual Period without the express written permission of Employer. Employer must take all vacation days at a time convenient to Employer, taking into account the exigencies of the Employer's business. Upon termination of Employee's employment with Employer, Employee will be entitled to vacation pay with respect to vacation days accrued but not taken, provided that Employee has not been terminated for Cause (as defined in Section 9). Upon termination of employment, if Employee has taken more vacation days than he is entitled during the current Vacation Accrual Period, a deduction shall be made from Employee's final paycheck in an amount equal to the excess of the value of vacation days taken over vacation days accrued. Except in the case of termination, vacation pay will not be paid in lieu of vacation days accrued but not taken.

9.   Termination by Employer. Employer may terminate this Agreement with or without Cause, as provided herein.

(a)   Termination by Employer with Cause. Employer may terminate Employee with Cause immediately and without notice. As used herein, "Cause" shall mean any of the following occurrences:

(i)   numerous recurring unexcused absences of Employee, within any two-month period;

(ii)   violation by Employee of any statute, regulation or ordinance applicable to, or the compliance with which is necessary for, operation of the business of Employer;

(iii)   breach by Employee of any of the provisions of this Agreement;

(iv)   willful disobedience or insubordination by Employee in connection with his duties as prescribed hereunder;

(v)   failure by Employee to satisfactorily and/or properly perform the duties and obligations required of him by Employer in connection with his employment or willful neglect by Employee in the performance of said duties and obligations;

(vi)   use by Employee during the term hereof of illegal substances which have a material adverse effect on the performance of the Employee's duties hereunder or upon the reputation, business, or goodwill of Employer; or any act of fraud or dishonesty by Employee of any material matters in connection with his employment hereunder; or any intentional act by Employee materially compromising Employee's ability to represent Employer with the public; or any intentional act or omission by Employee which substantially impairs Employer's business, goodwill or reputation;

(vii)   failure by Employee to follow acceptable, reasonable practices as prescribed by Employer or the Board of Directors or an executive officer of Employer for work safety or general conduct relating to the business of Employer or the premises of Employer;

(viii) failure by Employee to abide by the rules, policies, standards and regulations of Employer or those of its clients to which Employer is subject which are published or communicated to employees of Employer;

(ix)   Employee being convicted of a felony; or

(x)   Employee becoming by reason of injury or illness incapacitated or unable to perform his duties under this Agreement, which incapacity or inability continues more than one hundred eighty (180) consecutive days during any period of three hundred sixty (360) days except to the extent prohibited by the Family Medical Leave Act or other state or federal statute or regulation.

Notwithstanding the foregoing, no occurrence listed above as items (i), (iii), (v), (vii) and (viii) shall constitute Cause unless Employee receives written notice from Employer objecting to such occurrence, and Employee fails to remedy such occurrence within ten (10) days after the receipt of such written notice or subsequently repeats the same occurrence specified in such notice; provided, however, in no event shall Employer be required to give notice of or an opportunity to cure the occurrence of any of items (i), (iii), (v), (vii) or (viii) above more often than once for such an occurrence to constitute Cause hereunder. For items (ii), (iv), (vi), (ix) and (x), above, Employer may terminate Employee with Cause upon their occurrence without prior notice or opportunity to cure.

Upon Employee's termination with Cause, Employer shall be required to pay Employee compensation and benefits (and any unpaid expenses payable under Section 6) only through the effective date of termination. Sums due Employee for salary under Section 3 shall be prorated for the then current month through the date of termination. Any proration of compensation or benefits paid on a weekly basis shall be calculated based on a business week consisting of five (5) days and not seven (7) days. By way of example and not of limitation, two (2) weeks of vacation would be calculated as ten (10) business days.

(b)   Termination by Employer Without Cause. In the event that Employee's employment is terminated for reasons other than death or Cause, Employer shall be required (i) to give Employee the following written notice: (a) if Employee has been continuously employed for more than six (6) months but less than five (5) years, Employer shall provide Employee four (4) weeks' notice; and (b) if Employee has been continuously employed for more than five (5) complete and continuous years, Employer shall provide Employee one (1) week's notice for each complete year of service, subject to a maximum of twelve (12) weeks' notice; and (ii) to pay Employee any accrued but unpaid Base Salary for services rendered to the date of termination (and in all instances, exclusive of any bonus outstanding and payable to Employee by Employer) as well as any accrued but unpaid expenses required to be reimbursed under Section 7 and any vacation accrued to the date of termination.

(c)   Full Settlement. The post-termination payments provided for in this Section 9 shall be the only payments which Employer shall be obligated to make on account of the termination of Employee's employment, except all accrued and unused vacation benefits as of the termination date and after such termination, Employer shall not be obligated to make any other payments as damages or otherwise or provide any other benefits to or on behalf of Employee.

10.   Voluntary Termination. Employee may terminate this Agreement prior to the end of its term by delivering four (4) weeks' prior written notice to Employer. Employer may accept the proposed termination date or may set an earlier termination date by mailing or personally delivering notice of such earlier date to Employee. In the event Employee voluntarily terminates this Agreement, he will receive the salary due under Section 3 above through the effective date of termination and no other compensation or benefits, except all accrued and unused vacation benefits as of the termination date.

11.   Other Activities. Employee shall devote all of his working time and efforts during the Employer's normal business hours (reasonable vacations and sick leave excluded) to the business and affairs of Employer pursuant to this Agreement. Employee shall faithfully and diligently obey and act upon all reasonable and

lawful instructions and direction given to him by or on behalf of Employer. Employee's expenditure of reasonable amounts of time for personal, outside business, charitable and professional activities shall not be a breach of this Agreement, provided that such activities do not materially interfere with the services required to be rendered by Employee to Employer hereunder. The making of personal investments and the conduct of private business affairs shall not be prohibited hereunder, subject to Section 13 hereof.

12.   Confidential Information.

(a)   Definition. During the Term, Employer will disclose to Employee information, technical data and know-how regarding the business affairs, services and products of Employer as well as Employer's customers, which constitute Confidential Information. "Confidential Information" under this Agreement, whether or not specifically identified as confidential, shall consist of any and all proprietary information and proprietary data relating to Employer, and any derivative works thereof, including, by way of illustration and not limitation: (i) details of Employer's actual and potential clients, including lists of those persons and organizations; (ii) preferential terms of business and contracts between Employer and Its customers, including pricing information; (iii) research and development activities of Employer; (iv) Employer's plans for and details relating to product and service development; (v) proposals and tenders made by Employer to its customers' clients for proposed contracts or business; (vi) Employer's business plans, procedures and practices; (vii) financial information relating Employer; (viii) information and relationships with resources, suppliers and customers of Employer; and (ix) manufacturing processes, production specifications, techniques, methods, systems, trade secrets, discoveries, technology concepts, designs, drawings, schematics, plans, data, know-how, improvements, software programs (including without limitation, object code, source code, flow charts, algorithms and related documentation), listings, routines, manuals, products, structures, formulas, and personnel directories and files of the Employer, its employees, agents or customers. For the purposes of this Section 12, any and all proprietary information and proprietary date, as more fully described above, of any corporation in control of Employer (a "Parent") or any majority-owned subsidiary (a "Subsidiary") or any affiliate of Employer (an "Affiliate") shall be included within the definition of Confidential Information.

(b)   Protection of Confidential Information. All Confidential Information shall be the sole property of the Company and its assigns, and the Company shall be the sole owner of all patents, copyrights, intellectual property, inventions and other rights in connection therewith. Employee acknowledges that the Confidential Information is a special, valuable and unique asset of the Company, and Employee agrees at all times during the period of Employee's employment and thereafter to keep in confidence and trust all Confidential Information. Employee agrees that during the period of Employee's employment and at all times thereafter Employee will not directly or indirectly use the Confidential Information other than in the course of performing Employee's duties as an employee or officer of the Company, nor will Employee directly or indirectly disclose any Confidential Information to any person or entity, except in the course of performing such duties, and then only to those persons who are required to have such knowledge in connection with their work for the Company. Employee agrees that Confidential Information will not be disclosed by Employee to persons not in the employ of the Company without the prior written consent of the Company. As used herein, persons who are required to have such knowledge shall include, but not be limited to the Board of Directors of the Company and such officers, employees and agents of the Company or its affiliates to which such information is furnished in the normal course of business under established policies approved by the Company or its affiliates and such outside parties as are legally entitled to such information (other than as a result of action by Employee not previously approved or authorized by the Company or the Board of Directors of the Company) and customers and banking, lending, collection, and data-processing institutions or agencies in the course of maintaining ordinary business procedures of the Company. Employee will abide by the policies and regulations of the Company, as established from time to time, for the protection of Confidential Information. Employee agrees that Employee will not use any Confidential Information to contact or solicit employees or customers of the Company or any Parent, Subsidiary or Affiliate at any time during or after the termination of Employee's employment with the Company.

(c)   Limitations. The provisions of this Section 12 shall not be applicable to: (a) information which at the time of disclosure to Employee is a matter of public knowledge or in the public domain; or (b) information which, after disclosure to Employee, becomes public knowledge or in the public domain other than through a breach of this Agreement. Unless the Confidential Information shall be of the type hereinbefore set forth in the two immediately preceding sentences, Employee shall not use such Confidential Information for his own benefit or for a third party's or parties' benefit at any time. The obligations imposed upon Employee by this Section 12 shall survive the expiration or termination of this

Agreement. Concurrently with the execution of this Agreement, Employee shall execute a standard Proprietary Rights and Confidentiality Agreement in the form attached hereto as Exhibit B.

13. Covenant Not to Compete and Non-Solicitation by Employee.

(a) Competitive Activity. Employee covenants and agrees that at all times during his employment, Employee will not, directly or indirectly, engage in, assist, or have any active interest or involvement, whether as an employee, agent. consultant, independent contractor, joint venturer, associate, creditor, advisor, officer, director, stockholder (excluding holdings of less than five percent (5%) of the stock of another company for investment purposes only), partner, proprietor or any type of principal whatsoever, directly or indirectly, in any person, firm, or business entity, many business activities or with any business that competes with or is engaged in the same business as that conducted and carried on by Employer, without Employer's specific written consent to do so.

(b) Non-Solicitation. Employee covenants and agrees that at all times during his employment, Employee will not directly or indirectly, within the County _____: (1) induce, or attempt to induce, any customers of Employer or entities affiliated with Employer to patronize any similar business which competes with any material business of Employer; (2) canvass, solicit or accept, or attempt to canvass, solicit or accept, any similar business from any customer of Employer or entities affiliated with Employer; (3) request or advise any customers of Employer or entities affiliated with Employer to withdraw, curtail or cancel such customer's business with Employer; (4) disclose to any other person or entity the names or addresses of any of the customers of Employer or entities affiliated with Employer; or (5) individually or through any person or entity with which Employee is now or may hereafter become associated, cause, solicit, entice, or induce, or attempt to cause, solicit, entice or induce, any present or future employee of Employer or any entity affiliated with Employer to leave the employ of Employer, or such other entity to accept employment with, or compensation from, Employee or any such person or entity without the prior written consent of Employer.

(c)   Non-Disparagement. Employee covenants and agrees that Employee shall not engage in any pattern of conduct that involves the making or publishing of written or oral statements or remarks (including, without limitation, the repetition or distribution of derogatory rumors, allegations, negative reports or comments) which are disparaging, deleterious or damaging to the integrity, reputation or good will of Employer, its management, or of management of corporations affiliated with Employer.

(d)   Employee Claims. Employee represents and warrants that he has not complaint, claim or actions against Employer, or its officers, agents, directors, supervisors, employees or representatives with any state, federal or local agency or court and that Employee will not do so at any time hereafter unless arising from Employer's breach of this Agreement.

(e)   Inventions. Any and all inventions, discoveries, improvements, trade secrets, formulas, designs, layouts, circuits, techniques, software programs, processes, know-how, patent rights, letter patents, copyrights, trademarks, trade names and any applications therefore, in the U.S. and all other countries, or any other intellectual property, whether or not patentable and whether or not reduced to practice, and any and all rights and interest in, to and under the same, that are conceived, made, acquired, or possessed by Employee at any time during the term, whether alone or with other employees, shall become the exclusive property of Employer and shall at all times and for all purposes be regarded as acquired and held by Employee in a fiduciary capacity for the sole benefit of Employer, and Employee shall forthwith disclose the doing of and all details of the same to Employer, and Employee hereby assigns and agrees to assign the same to Employer without further compensation. Employee agrees to promptly make all disclosures, execute all applications, assignments or other instruments and perform all acts whatsoever necessary or desired by Employer to vest and confirm in it, its successors, assigns and nominees, fully and completely, all rights and interests created or contemplated by this Section 13. Concurrently with the execution of this Agreement, Employee shall execute a standard Proprietary Rights and Confidentiality Agreement in the form attached hereto as Exhibit B.

14.   Employer Property. All products, records, designs, patents, plans, data, manuals, field guides, catalogs, brochures, minutes, memoranda, correspondence, reports, machinery, devices, lists and other documents or property delivered to Employee by or on behalf of Employer or a Parent, Subsidiary, Affiliate or customer of Employer (including, but not limited to, Employer's customers solicited by Employee), and all records and documents compiled by Employee which pertain to the business of Employer or a Parent, Subsidiary or Affiliate shall be and remain the property of Employer and be subject at all times to its discretion and control. Employee shall promptly deliver to a designated representative of Employer all such property, as well as any and all correspondence with customers and representatives, reports, records, charts, advertising materials, and other materials, and property in his possession or control which belong to Employer upon termination of Employee's employment.

15.   Representations of Employee.

(a)   Employee represents that to the best of his knowledge he is not the subject of any pending or threatened claim which involves any criminal or governmental proceedings, or allegations of misfeasance, and that he has not been charged nor threatened to be charged by any governmental or administrative body with violation of law except for minor traffic violations and similar charges.

(b)   Employee represents and warrants that he is not prohibited from acting in any capacity for Employer by virtue of the operation of any non-competition or similar agreement with any prior employer, or by any applicable statutes, regulations or ordinances or any other applicable law or by the rules and regulations of the U.S. Securities and Exchange Commission or any national securities exchange, and that his acting in any capacity for Employer will not subject Employer to claims or materially impair the license status of Employer or its affiliates or any business operated by Employer or its affiliates.

16.   Defense of Claims. Employee agrees that during the Term, and at all reasonable times thereafter, he will cooperate with Employer in the defense of any claim that may be made against Employer or any affiliates, to the extent that such claims may relate to services performed by Employee for Employer or its affiliates, in connection with such claim: (i) if Employee is required to travel more than one hundred (100) miles from his home, Employer agrees to reimburse Employee for all of his reasonable out-of-pocket expenses associated with such travel and, to the extent reasonably practicable, to provide Employee with notice of at least ten (10) days prior to the date on which such travel is required; and (ii) if Employee is no longer employed by Employer, to compensate Employee at a reasonable rate.

17. Injunction and Other Relief.

(a) Injunctions. Both parties hereto recognize that the services to be rendered under this Agreement by Employee are special, unique and of extraordinary character, and that in the event of the breach by Employee of any of the terms and conditions of this Agreement to be performed by him, or in the event Employee performs services for any person, firm or corporation in violation of Section 13, or if Employee shall breach the provisions of this Agreement with respect to Confidential Information, then Employer shall be entitled, if it so elects, in addition to all other remedies available to it under this Agreement or at law or in equity, to affirmative injunctive or other equitable relief, and Employee waives (and shall execute such documents as may be necessary to further evidence such waiver) any requirement that Employer secure or post any bond in connection with such injunctive or other equitable relief.

(b) Mandatory Arbitration. The Employee and Employer agree that any claim, controversy or dispute between the Employee and Employer (including without limitation its affiliates, officers, employees, representatives, or agents) arising out of or relating to this Agreement, the employment of the Employee, the cessation of employment of the Employee, or any matter relating to the foregoing shall be submitted to and settled by arbitration in a forum of the American Arbitration Association ("AAA") located in _____ County in the State of California and conducted in accordance with the National Rules for the Resolution of Employment Disputes. In such arbitration: (i) each arbitrator shall agree to treat as confidential evidence and other information presented by the parties to the same extent as Confidential Information under this Agreement must be held confidential by the Employee, (ii) the arbitrators shall have no authority to amend or modify any of the terms of this Agreement, and (iii) the arbitrators shall have ten business days from the closing statements or submission of post-hearing briefs by the parties to render their decision. Any arbitration award shall be final and binding upon the parties, and any court, state or federal, having jurisdiction may enter a judgment on the award. The foregoing requirement to arbitrate claims, controversies, and disputes applies to all claims or demands by the Employee, including without limitation any rights or claims the Employee may have under the Age Discrimination in Employment Act of 1967 (which prohibits age discrimination in employment), Title VII of the Civil Rights Act of 1964 (which prohibits discrimination in employment based on race, color, national origin, religion, sex or pregnancy), the Americans with Disabilities Act of 1991 (which prohibits discrimination in employment against qualified persons with a disability), the Equal Pay Act (which prohibits paying men and women unequal pay for equal work) or any other federal, state, or local laws or regulations pertaining to the Employee's employment or the termination of the Employee's employment.

(c)   Recovery of Legal Fees. If one of the parties to this Agreement (the "Plaintiff") should bring a proceeding against the other party (the "Defendant") in connection with an alleged breach or threatened breach of this Agreement, and if such proceeding is ultimately resolved by an order or a judgment in favor of the Defendant, by a voluntary discontinuance with prejudice by the Plaintiff, or by an arbitration decision wholly in favor of the Defendant, the Plaintiff will, upon presentation by the Defendant of appropriate evidence of the amount and nature of the expense incurred, reimburse the Defendant in an amount equal to the lesser of:

(i)   the cost of all reasonable legal fees actually incurred by the Defendant in connection with such litigation or arbitration; or

(ii) $100,000.

18.   <u>Stipulation</u>. Employee hereby specifically acknowledges, agrees, stipulates and represents to Employer that:

(a)   Employee has received adequate and sufficient consideration for entering into this Agreement including the above-referenced compensation;

(b)   the execution and delivery of this Agreement and the performance hereunder do not and shall not constitute a violation of any covenants of non-competition, trade secrecy, or confidentiality to which Employee is a party;

(c)   the covenants of Employee contained in Section 12 and Section 13 of this Agreement are in consideration of the promise of Employer to provide Confidential Information (including trade secrets) to Employee and are necessary to protect Employer's interests in such Confidential Information, as well as Employer's business, goodwill and other business interests;

(d)   Employer will suffer great loss and irreparable harm if Employee competes directly or indirectly with Employer;

(e)   the temporal, geographic and other restrictions contained in this Agreement are in all respects reasonable and necessary to protect the business, goodwill, Confidential Information, trade secrets, prospects and other business interests of Employer; and

(f)   the enforcement of this Agreement will not work an undue or unfair hardship on Employee or otherwise be oppressive to him.

19.   <u>Variation in Terms and Conditions of Employment</u>. Employer reserves the right to vary the terms and conditions of employment by giving Employee thirty (30) days' prior notice in writing of the nature of the variation. If for whatever reason it

shall not be possible for Employer to notify Employee in advance of any variation to these terms and conditions of employment in the manner set forth in the preceding sentence, then Employer shall notify Employee in writing of the nature of the variation within one month of its coming into effect.

20. <u>Severability</u>. In the event that any of the provisions of this Agreement shall be held invalid or unenforceable by any court of competent jurisdiction, such invalidity or unenforceability shall not affect the remainder of this Agreement and same shall be construed as if such invalid or unenforceable provisions had never been a part hereof. If a court of competent jurisdiction determines that the length of time, geographical restrictions or any other restriction, or portion thereof, set forth in this Agreement is overly restrictive and unenforceable, the parties agree that the court shall reduce or modify such restrictions to those which it deems reasonable and enforceable under the circumstances, and as so reduced or modified, the parties hereto agree that the restrictions of this Agreement shall remain in full force and effect. In the event there is a breach by Employer or Employee of any other provision of this Agreement, the covenants contained in Sections 12 and 13 shall remain in full force and effect.

21. <u>Waiver</u>. The waiver by either party of a breach or violation of any provision of this Agreement shall not operate as or be construed to be a waiver of any subsequent or continuing breach hereof. The failure of any party to insist upon strict adherence to any provision of this Agreement on one or more occasions shall not be considered a waiver.

22. <u>Notices</u>. Any notices provided for in this Agreement shall be given in writing and transmitted by personal delivery or prepaid first class registered or certified U.S. mail addressed as follows:

Employer: _____

_____

_____

With a copy to: _____

_____

_____

_____

Employee: _____

_____

_____

23. <u>Successors to Employer</u>. Except as otherwise provided herein, this Agreement shall inure to the benefit of Employer and any successor of Employer, including, without limitation, any entity or entities acquiring directly or indirectly all or substantially all of the assets or business of Employer whether by merger, consolidation, sale or otherwise (and such successor shall thereafter be deemed Employer for the purposes of this Agreement), but shall not otherwise be assignable by Employer.

24. <u>Transfer and Assignment</u>. This agreement is personal as to Employee and shall not be assigned or transferred by Employee without the prior written consent of Employer.

25. <u>Governing Law</u>. This Agreement shall be governed by and construed in accordance with the laws of the State of California, without regard to applicable conflicts of law.

26. <u>Choice of Forum</u>. The parties hereto agree that in the event that any legal suits, actions or proceedings arising out of this Agreement are instituted by any party hereto, such suits, actions or proceedings shall be instituted only in the state or federal courts In the County of _____ in the State of California. The parties hereto do hereby consent to the jurisdiction of such courts and waive any objection which they may, now or hereafter have to the venue of any such suits, actions or proceedings; <u>provided</u>, <u>however</u>, that any party hereto shall have the right to institute proceedings in another jurisdiction if the purpose of such proceedings is to enforce or realize upon any final court judgment arising out of this Agreement.

27. <u>Consent to Service</u>. Service of any and all process which may be served on any party hereto in any suit, action or proceeding related to this Agreement may be made by registered or certified mail, return receipt requested, to Employee or Employer at their respective addresses for notice as set forth in Section 24 and service so made shall be taken and held to be valid personal service upon such party by any party to this Agreement on whose behalf such service is made.

28. <u>Entire Agreement</u>. This Agreement constitutes the entire agreement between the parties, superseding all prior understandings, arrangements and agreements, whether oral or written, and may not be amended except by a writing signed by the parties hereto. As used herein, unless the context otherwise indicates, the term "this Agreement" means the Agreement executed to be effective as of the Effective Date and any written amendments thereof.

29. <u>Counterparts</u>. This Agreement may be executed in counterparts, each of which shall be deemed to be an original, but both of which together shall constitute one and the same instrument.

IN WITNESS WHEREOF, Employer has, by its appropriate officers, executed this Agreement and Employee has executed this Agreement on the _____ day of _____ , 200_, to be effective as of the Effective Date.

NEW ERA HEALTH SYSTEM

By: _____

Its: _____

EMPLOYEE

Name: _____

Exhibit A

Employee Duties

The employee duties shall be based around, but not limited to:

_____

_____

_____

_____

_____

_____

_____

_____

_____

_____

_____

_____

_____

_____

_____

_____

_____

_____

_____

_____

_____

_____

_____

_____

_____

_____

_____

_____

Exhibit B

Proprietary Rights and Confidentiality Agreement

THIS PROPRIETARY RIGHTS AND CONFIDENTIAL-ITY AGREEMENT (this "Agreement") is effective as of _____, 200_ (the "Effective Date"), by and between New Era Health System, a California corporation (the "Company"), and _____, a resident of _____, _____, California ("Employee"), under the following terms and conditions:

R E C I T A L S:

A.   Employee is or is about to become an employee or officer of the Company;

B.   During the course of Employee's employment with the Company, Employee will have access to important confidential and proprietary information and trade secrets of the Company and its suppliers and customers, and

C.   Employee voluntarily enters into this Agreement for the purpose of providing for and confirming the Company's ownership of all Inventions (as defined herein), and to set forth the understanding and agreement of Employee with the Company relating to the Company's Confidential Information (as defined herein).

NOW, THEREFORE, in consideration of Employees initial or continuing employment by the Company as an officer and/or employee and the compensation received therefore, and for other good and valuable consideration, the receipt and sufficiency of which is hereby specifically acknowledged, Employee hereby agrees with the Company as follows:

2.   Employment Relationship.

Employee acknowledges that Employee's employment creates a relationship of confidence and trust between Employee and the Company with respect to all Confidential Information (as defined herein) of the Company.

3.   Confidential Information.

(a)   Definition. Confidential Information under this Agreement whether or not specifically identified as confidential, shall consist of any and all proprietary information and proprietary data relating to the Company, and any derivative works thereof, including, by way of illustration and not limitation: (i) details of the Company's actual and potential clients, including lists of those persons and organizations; (ii) preferential terms of business and contracts between the Company and its customers, including pricing information; (iii) research and development activities of the Company, (iv) the Company's plans for and details relating to product and service development; (v) proposals and tenders made by the Company to its customers' clients for proposed contract or business; (vi) the Company's business plans, procedures and practices; (vii) financial information relating to the Company; (viii) information and relationships with resources, suppliers and customers of the Company; and (ix) manufacturing processes, production specifications, techniques, methods, systems, trade secrets, discoveries, technology, concepts, designs, drawings, schematics, plans, data, know-how, improvements, software programs (including without limitation, object code, source code, flow charts, algorithms and related documentation), listings, routines, manuals, products, structures, formulas, and personnel directories and files of the Company, its employees, agents or customers. For the purposes of this Section 2, any and all proprietary information and proprietary data, as more fully described above, of any corporation in control of the Company (a "Parent") or any majority-owned subsidiary (a "Subsidiary") or any Affiliate of the Company (an "Affiliate") shall be included within the definition of Confidential Information.

(b)   Protection of Confidential Information. All Confidential Information shall be the sole property of the Company and its assigns, and the Company shall be the sole owner of all patents, copyrights, intellectual property, inventions and other rights in connection therewith. Employee acknowledges that the Confidential Information is a special, valuable and unique asset of the Company, and Employee agrees at all times during the period of Employee's employment and thereafter to keep in confidence and trust all Confidential Information. Employee agrees that during the period of Employee's employment and at all times thereafter, Employee will not directly or indirectly use the Confidential Information other than in the course of performing Employee's duties as an employee or officer of the Company, nor will Employee directly or indirectly disclose any Confidential Information to any person or entity, except in the course of performing such duties, and then only to those persons who are required to have such knowledge in connection with their work for the Company. Employee agrees that Confidential Information will not be disclosed by Employee to persons not in the employ of the Company without the prior written consent of the Company. As used herein, persons who are required to have such knowledge shall include, but not be limited to, the Board of Directors of the Company and such officers, employees and agents of the Company or its affiliates to which such information is furnished in the normal course of business under established policies approved by the Company or its affiliates and such outside parties as are legally entitled to such information (other than as a result of action by Employee not previously approved or authorized by the Company or the Board of Directors of the Company) and customers and banking, lending, collection and data processing institutions or agencies in the course of maintaining ordinary business procedures of the Company. Employee will abide by the policies and regulations of the Company, as established from time to time, for the protection of Confidential Information. Employee agrees that Employee will not use any Confidential Information to contact or solicit employees or customers of the Company or any Parent, Subsidiary or Affiliate at any time during or after the termination of Employee's employment with the Company.

(c)   Limitations. The provisions of this Section 2 shall not be applicable to: (a) information which at the time of disclosure to Employee is a matter of public knowledge or in the public domain; or (b) information which, after disclosure to Employee, becomes public knowledge or in the public domain other than through a breach of this Agreement. Unless the Confidential Information shall be of the type hereinbefore set forth in the two immediately preceding sentences, Employee shall not use such Confidential Information for his own benefit or for a third party's or parties' benefit at any time. The obligations imposed upon Employee by this Section 2 shall survive the expiration or termination of this Agreement.

4.   Return of Materials.

All products, records, designs, patents, plans, data, manuals, field guides, catalogs, brochures, minutes, memoranda, correspondence, reports, machinery, devices, lists and other documents or property delivered to Employee by or on behalf of the Company or a Parent, Subsidiary, Affiliate or customer of the Company (including, but not limited to, the Company's customers solicited by Employee), and all records and documents compiled by Employee which pertain to the business of the Company or a Parent, Subsidiary or Affiliate shall be and remain the property of the Company and be subject at all times to its discretion and control. Employee shall promptly deliver to a designated representative of the Company all such property, as well as any and all correspondence with customers and representatives, reports, records, charts, advertising materials, and other materials, and property in his possession or control which belong to the Company upon termination of Employee's employment.

5.   Covenant Not to Compete and Non-Solicitation by Employee.

(a)   Competitive Activity. Employee covenants and agrees that at all times during his employment, Employee will not, directly or indirectly, engage in, assist, or have any active interest or involvement, whether as an employee, agent, consultant, independent contractor, joint venturer, associate, creditor, advisor, officer, director, stockholder (excluding holdings of less than five percent (5%) of the stock of another company for investment purposes only), partner, proprietor or any type of principal whatsoever, directly or indirectly, in any person, firm, or business entity, in any business activities or with any business that competes with or is engaged in the same business as that conducted and carried on by the Company, without the Company's specific written consent to do so.

(b)   Non-Solicitation. Employee covenants and agrees that at all times during his employment, Employee will not directly or indirectly, within the County of _____ in the State of California: (1) induce, or attempt to induce, any customers of the Company or entities affiliated with the Company to patronize any similar business which competes with any material business of the Company; (2) canvass, solicit or accept, or attempt to canvass, solicit or accept, any similar business from any customer of the Company or entities affiliated with the Company; (3) request or advise any customers of the Company or entities affiliated with the Company to withdraw, curtail or cancel such customer's business with the Company; (4) disclose to any other person or entity the names or addresses of any of the customers of the Company or entities affiliated with the Company; or (5) individually or through any person or entity with which Employee is now or may hereafter become associated, cause, solicit, entice, or induce, or attempt to cause, solicit, entice or induce, any present or future employee of the Company or any entity affiliated with the Company to leave the employ of the Company, or such other entity to accept with, or compensation from, Employee or any such person or entity without the prior written consent of the Company.

(c) <u>Non-Disparagement.</u> Employee covenants and agrees that Employee shall not engage in any pattern of conduct that involves the making or publishing of written or oral statements or remarks (including, without limitation, the repetition or distribution of derogatory rumors, allegations, negative reports or comments) which are disparaging, deleterious or damaging to the integrity, reputation or good will of the Company, its management, or of management of corporations affiliated with the Company.

6.   <u>Disclosure to Company; Inventions as Sole Property of Company</u>.

(a)   Employee agrees to promptly disclose to the Company any and all inventions, discoveries, improvements, trade secrets, formulas, designs, layouts, circuits, techniques, software programs, processes, know-how, patent rights, letter patents, copyrights, trademarks, trade names and any applications therefore, in the U.S. and all other countries, or any other intellectual property, whether or not patentable and whether or not reduced to practice, conceived or learned by Employee, either alone or jointly with others, during the period of Employee's employment which relate in any manner to the actual or anticipated business, work, research or investigations of the Company or any Parent, Subsidiary or Affiliate or which result, to any extent, from the use of the Company's premises or property (the foregoing being hereinafter collectively referred to as "Inventions").

(b)   Employee acknowledges and agrees that all the Inventions shall be the sole property of the Company or any other entity designated by it, and Employee hereby assigns to the Company Employee's entire right and interest in and to all the Inventions. The Company or any other entity designated by it shall be the sole owner of all domestic and foreign patents, patent rights, copyrights, mask work rights and other proprietary rights pertaining to the Inventions. Employee further agrees, as to all the Inventions, to assist the Company in every way (at the Company's expense) to obtain and, from time to time, enforce patents on the Inventions in any and all countries. To that end, by way of illustration but not limitation, Employee will testify in any suit or other proceeding involving any of the Inventions, execute all documents which the Company reasonably determines to be necessary or convenient for use in applying for and obtaining patents, copyrights, mask work rights or other enforceable rights with respect thereto and enforcing same, and execute all necessary assignments thereof to the Company or persons designated by it. Employee's obligation to assist the Company in obtaining and enforcing patents, copyright, mask work rights or other enforceable rights with respect to the Inventions in any and all countries shall continue beyond the termination of Employee's employment, but the Company shall compensate Employee at a reasonable rate after such termination for time actually spent by Employee at the Company's request on such assistance.

(c)   Employee acknowledges and agrees that all software developed by Employee while Employee is performing any services for the Company, any Parent, Subsidiary or Affiliate, and all original materials submitted or prepared by Employee as part of the software or as part of the process of creating the software, including, but not limited to, source code, object code, listings, printouts, documentation, notes, flow charts and programming aides, shall be the property of the Company, or the Parent, Subsidiary, Affiliate or any other person who the Company, any Parent, any Subsidiary or any Affiliate has agreed shall have the ownership thereof. No rights in any such software are reserved to Employee. Employee further agrees to forebear from asserting all moral rights or comparable rights that Employee may have in such materials, including without limitation, any right to prevent modification of the materials, any rights to receive attribution of authorship, or any right to control the materials.

(d)   Notwithstanding the provisions of subparagraphs (a)–(c) above, as provided in Section 2870 of the California Labor Code, a copy of which accompanies this Agreement as Exhibit B, this Section 5 does not apply to any Inventions:

That the Employee developed entirely on his own time without using the Company's equipment supplies, facilities, or trade secret information except for those inventions that either:

(i)   Relate at the time of conception or reduction to practice of the invention to the Company's business, or actual or demonstrably anticipated research or development of the Company; or

(ii)   Result from any work performed by Employee for the company.

(e)   Employee agrees to keep and maintain adequate and current records of all Inventions made, conceived, developed or perfected during the period of Employee's employment and that such records shall be available to, and remain the sole property of, the Company at all times; provided, however, that if Employee believes that any Invention meets the criteria of subparagraph (d)above, Employee will advise the Company promptly of such invention and provide to the Company in writing evidence necessary to substantiate such belief. The Company will keep in confidence and not disclose to third parties without Employee's consent any Confidential Information disclosed in writing to the Company relating to inventions that qualify fully under the provisions of Section 2970 of the California Labor Code.

7.   <u>List of Prior Inventions</u>.

All inventions, if any, which Employee made prior to Employee's employment by the Company are excluded from the scope of this Agreement. As a matter of record, Employee has set forth on Exhibit A attached hereto a complete list of all inventions, discoveries or improvements relating in any way to the business or proposed business of the Company or any Parent, Subsidiary or Affiliate which have been made by Employee, alone or jointly with others, prior to Employee's employment with the Company. Employee represents and warrants that such list is complete and that to the best of Employee's knowledge, the removal of inventions listed thereon from the operation of this Agreement will not materially affect Employees ability to perform the duties for which Employee is employed by the Company.

8.   <u>No Breach of Other Agreements.</u>

Employee represents and warrants that Employee's performance of all the terms of this Agreement and Employee's performance of all duties as an employee or officer of the Company or any Parent, Subsidiary or Affiliate which Employee may reasonably foresee do not and will not breach any agreement to keep in confidence proprietary information acquired by Employee in confidence or in trust prior to Employee's employment with the Company, and Employee agrees not to enter into any agreement either written or oral in conflict with this representation and warranty.

9.   <u>Indemnification.</u>

Employee shall indemnify the Company and any Parent, Subsidiary or Affiliate, and hold each of them harmless, from and against any and all claims, losses, damages, judgments and liabilities attributable to Employee's breach of any representation, warranty or covenant of Employee under this Agreement and shall reimburse each of them for all of its costs, expenses and attorneys' fees paid or incurred in connection therewith.

10.   <u>Injunction.</u>

Employee agrees that it would be difficult to measure damage to the Company from any breach by Employee of the covenants set forth in Paragraphs 2, 3, 4 and 5 herein, that injury to the Company from any such breach would be impossible to calculate, and that monetary damages would therefore be an inadequate remedy for any such breach. Accordingly, Employee agrees that if Employee shall breach Paragraphs 2, 3, 4 and 5 hereof, the Company shall be entitled, in addition to all other remedies it may have, to injunctions or other appropriate orders to restrain any such breach by Employee without showing or proving any actual damage sustained by the Company.

11. <u>Advertising.</u>

Employee agrees that the Company may use Employee's name or photograph to its commercial interests in advertising its products or services or in general publicity. Photographs, which may be taken of Employee by the Company in the course of Employee's work, will remain the sole and exclusive property of the Company.

12. <u>Effective Date; No Term of Employment.</u>

This Agreement shall be effective as of the first date of Employee's employment by the Company. This Agreement does not create an employment relationship for a term or limit in any way the rights of Employee or the Company to terminate Employee's employment at any time for any reason whatsoever, with or without cause. This Agreement is not an employment contract.

13. <u>No Third Party Beneficiaries.</u>

The parties hereto do not intend to create any third party beneficiaries of their agreement hereunder, and no person or entity other than such parties, any Parent, Subsidiary and any Affiliate and their respective successors, heirs and permitted assigns, shall have any rights under this Agreement.

14. <u>General.</u>

(a) To the extent that any of the agreements set forth herein, or any word, phrase, clause, or sentence thereof shall be found to be illegal or unenforceable for any reason, such agreement, word, clause, phrase or sentence shall be modified or deleted in such a manner so as to make the agreement as modified legal and enforceable under applicable laws, and the balance of the agreements or parts thereof, shall not be effected thereby, the balance being construed as severable and independent.

(b) This Agreement shall be binding upon Employee and Employee's heirs, executors, assigns, and administrators and shall inure to the benefit of the Company, its successors and assigns and any Parent, Subsidiary or Affiliate.

(c) This Agreement may be signed in two counterparts, each of which shall be deemed an original and which together shall constitute one instrument.

(d) This Agreement shall be governed by the laws of the State of California without regard to any principles governing conflicts of laws.

(e) In any litigation concerning this Agreement, the prevailing party shall be entitled to receive its reasonable attorneys' fees, costs and related expenses.

(f) This Agreement represents the entire agreement between Employee and the Company with respect to the subject matter hereof, superseding all previous oral or written communications, representations or agreements. This Agreement may be modified only by a duly authorized and executed written agreement.

IN WITNESS WHEREOF, this Agreement has been executed by Employee and the Company as of the date first above written.

EMPLOYEE

_____

NEW ERA HEALTH SYSTEM

_____

By: _____

Title: _____

CAUTION TO EMPLOYEE: This Agreement affects important rights. DO NOT sign it unless you have read it carefully and are satisfied that you understand it completely.

Exhibit A

       The following is a complete list of all inventions, discoveries or improvements relating in any way to the Company's business or Employee's existing or proposed employment by the Company which have been made by Employee prior to Employee's employment with the Company.

<u>Employee's Initials</u>

_____ None

_____ As listed below (use additional sheets if necessary):

_____

_____

_____

_____

_____

_____ additional sheets attached.

Acknowledged:

_____

By: _____

Dated: _____

Exhibit B

Inventions Made by an Employee

§2870. Employment agreements: assignment of rights

(a)   Any Provision in an employment agreement which provides that an employee shall assign, or offer to assign, any of his or her rights in an Invention to his or her employer shall not apply to an invention that the employee developed entirely on his or her own time without using the employer's equipment, supplies, facilities, or trade secret information except for those inventions that either:

(1) Relate at the time of conception or reduction to practice of the invention to the employer's business, or actual or demonstrably anticipated research or development of the employer, or

(2) Result from any work performed by the employee for the employer.

(d)   To the extent a provision in an employment agreement purports to require an employee to assign an invention otherwise excluded from being required to be assigned under subdivision (a), the provision is against the public policy of this state and is unenforceable.

§2871. Conditions of employment or continued employment; disclosure of inventions

No employer shall require a provision made void and unenforceable by Section 2870 as a condition of employment or continued employment. Nothing in this article shall be construed to forbid or restrict the right of an employer to provide in contracts of employment for disclosure, provided that any such disclosures be received in confidence, of all of the employee's inventions made solely or jointly with others during the term of his or her employment, a review process by the employer to determine such issues as may arise, and for full title to certain patents and inventions to be in the United States, as required by contracts between the employer and the United States or any of its agencies.

§2872. Notice to employee; burden of proof

If an employment agreement entered into after January 1, 1980, contains a provision requiring the employee to assign or offer to assign any of his or her rights in any invention to his or her employer, the employer must also, at the time the agreement is made, provide a written notification to the employee that the agreement does not apply to an invention which qualifies fully under the provisions of Section 2870. In any suit or action arising thereunder, the burden of proof shall be on the employee claiming the benefits of its provisions.

New ERA Health System Change in Control Plan

SECTION 1

Introduction

1.1.   Purpose. New Era Health System, a California nonprofit corporation, ("New Era"), has established the New Era Health System Change In Control Plan (the "Plan") to enable New Era and its Subsidiaries (as such term is defined in Section 1.3 hereof) (collectively, the "Company") to provide severance benefits to eligible executive or management employees whose employment is terminated following a Change in Control of the Company. It is the intent of the Company that the Plan, as set forth herein, constitutes an "employee welfare benefit plan" within the meaning of Section 3(1) of the Employee Retirement Income Act of 1974 ("ERISA") and complies with the applicable requirements of ERISA.

1.2.   Effective Date, Plan Year The "Effective Date" of the Plan is November 1, 2001. A "Plan Year" is the 12-month period beginning on January 1 and ending on the following December 31.

1.3.   Employers. Any Subsidiary of New Era employing an employee who has been designated as a Participant by the Committee shall be deemed to have adopted the Plan. A "Subsidiary" of New Era is any corporation more than 50 percent of the voting memberships or stock of which is owned, directly or indirectly, by New Era.

1.4.   Administration. The Plan is administered by the Executive Compensation Committee of the Board of Directors (the "Committee"). The Committee, from time to time, may adopt such rules and regulations as may be necessary or desirable for the proper and efficient administration of the Plan and as are consistent with the terms of the Plan. The Committee, from time to time, may also appoint such individuals to act as its representatives as the Committee considers necessary or desirable for the effective administration of the Plan. Any notice or document required to be given or filed with the committee will be properly given or filed if delivered or mailed, by registered mail, postage prepaid, to the Committee at [address].

SECTION 2

Participation

The Committee shall designate from time to time those employees of the Company employed in an executive or management position who shall participate in the plan (a "Participant"). An employee who has been so designated shall participate by signing an agreement with the Company, substantially in the form attached hereto as Exhibit A ("Participant's Agreement"), which shall specify the benefits the Participant is entitled to receive should the Participant's employment terminate following a Change in Control of the Company and the terms and conditions under which those benefits will be provided. A Participant's Agreement implements and forms a part of the Plan as respects the Participant's participation in the Plan. To the extent there are any inconsistencies between the Plan document and a Participant's Agreement, the terms of the Participant's Agreement shall be controlling. No employee other those designated by the Committee shall be eligible to participate in the Plan.

SECTION 3

Plan Benefits

3.1.   Benefits Following a Change in Control. If a Participant's employment with the Company terminates within twelve (12) to twenty-four (24) months following a Change in Control, as specified in a Participant's Agreement, the Participant shall be entitled to the benefits specified in the Participant's Agreement and such benefits shall be paid at such time, in such manner and subject to such conditions as are specified in the Agreement. A Participant's entitlement to benefits as specified in the Participant's Agreement shall depend upon whether the Participant's termination is voluntary or involuntary and whether for Cause (as such term is defined below), if involuntary, or for Good Reason (as such term is defined below), if voluntary.

3.2.   Non-Solicitation. In consideration for the benefits provided for under a Participant's Agreement, the Participant shall agree that during the 24-month period following the Participant's date of termination (the "Severance Period"), the Participant will not, without the prior written consent of Company, alone or in association with others, solicit on behalf of the Participant, or any Competing Business, any employee of Company for employment with a Competing Business. A Competing Business shall be defined to be any business engaged in any business and activities engaged in by the Company.

If a Participant fails to comply with the restrictions of this subsection 3.2 and the Participant's Agreement, participation in the Plan shall immediately terminate and the Participant shall forfeit any remaining unpaid benefits.

3.3.   Change in Control. For purposes of the Plan a "Change in Control" shall have occurred if: (a) any "Person" (as such term is used in Sections 13(d) and 14(d) of the Securities Exchange Act of 1934, as amended ("Exchange Act") other than

New Era), becomes the "beneficial owner" (as such term is defined in rule 13d-3 under the Exchange Act), directly or indirectly, of memberships of New Era representing 20% or more of the combined voting power of _____'s then outstanding memberships; (b) during any period of not more than 24 months, individuals who at the beginning of such period constitute the Board of Directors of New Era, and any new director (other than a director designated by a Person who has entered into an agreement with New Era to effect a transaction described in paragraph (a), (c), or (d) of this Section 3) whose election by the board or nomination for election by _____'s members was approved by a vote of at least two-thirds of the directors then still in office who either were directors at the beginning of the period or whose election or nomination for election was previously so approved, cease for any reason to constitute at least a majority thereof; (c) the Board of Directors of New Era approves a merger or consolidation of New Era or New Era Hospital Association (the "Association") with any other corporation, other than (i) a merger or consolidation which would result in the voting memberships of New Era outstanding immediately prior thereto continuing to represent (by being converted into voting memberships of the surviving entity) more than 60% of the combined voting power of the voting memberships of New Era or such surviving entity outstanding immediately after such merger or consolidation, or (ii) a merger or consolidation effected to implement a recapitalization of New Era (or similar transaction) in which no Person acquires more than 20% of the combined voting power of New Era's then outstanding memberships; or (d) the Board of Directors of New Era approves a plan of complete liquidation of New Era or the Association or an agreement for the sale or disposition by New Era or the Association of all or substantially all of its assets (or any transaction having a similar effect).

3.4. Terminations for Cause and Good Reason. A Participant will be considered to have been terminated for "Cause" if the termination is by reason of the Participant willfully engaging in conduct demonstrably and materially injurious to the Company, the Participant being convicted of or confessing to a crime involving dishonesty or moral turpitude or the Participant's willful and continued failure for a significant period of time to perform the Participant's duties after a demand for substantial performance has been delivered to the Participant by the Board of Directors of New Era which demand specifically identifies the manner in which the Board believes that the Participant has not substantially performed his duties. A Participant's termination shall be considered to have been for "Good Reason" if the Participant's termination is by reason of the occurrence of any of the following events within the twelve (12) to twenty-four (24) month period specified in a Participant's Agreement following a Change in Control without the Participant's express written consent:

(a)   any change in the Participant's title, authorities, responsibilities (including reporting responsibilities) which, in the Participant's judgment, represents an adverse change; the assignment to the Participant of any duties or work responsibilities which, in Participant's reasonable judgment, are inconsistent with such title, authorities or responsibilities; or any removal of the Participant from, or failure to reappoint or reelect him/her to any of such positions, except if any such changes are because of disability, retirement or Cause;

(b)   a reduction in or failure to pay any portion of the Participant's annual base salary as in effect on the date of the Change in Control or as the same may be increased from time to time thereafter;

(c)   the failure by the Company to provide the Participant with compensation and benefits (including, without limitation, incentive, bonus and other compensation plans and any vacation, medical, hospitalization, life insurance, dental or disability benefit plan), or cash compensation in lieu thereof, which are, in the aggregate, no less favorable than those provided by the Company to the Participant immediately prior to the occurrence of the Change in Control;

(d)   any breach by the Company of any provision of a Participant's Agreement; and

(e)   the failure of the Company to obtain a satisfactory agreement from any successor or assign of the Company to assume and agree to perform the Participant's Agreement.

SECTION 4

Payment of Benefits

4.1.   <u>Agreement Governs</u>. Any benefits under the Plan shall be payable at such time, and pursuant to the terms and conditions of each Participant's Agreement.

4.2.   <u>Form of Payment</u>. Subject to the terms of a Participant's Agreement, benefits shall be paid in equal installments according to the Company's normal payroll schedule. In the event of a Participant's death before the Participant receives all benefits to which he otherwise would be entitled under the Plan, payment shall be made to the Participant's beneficiary in installments or a lump sum, as determined by the Committee.

4.3.   <u>Designation of Beneficiary</u>. By signing a form furnished by the Committee, each Participant may designate any person or persons to whom his benefits are to be paid if he dies before he receives all of his benefits. A beneficiary designation form will be effective only when the form is filed with the Committee while the Participant is still alive and will cancel all beneficiary designation forms previously filed by the Participant with respect to this Plan. If a deceased Participant has failed to designate a beneficiary as provided above, or if the designated beneficiary predeceases the participant, payment of the Participant's benefits shall be made to the Participant's estate. If a designated beneficiary dies before complete payment of any benefits attributable to a Participant, remaining benefits shall be paid to the beneficiary's estate.

SECTION 5

Financing Plan Benefits

All benefits payable under the Plan shall be paid directly by the Company out of general assets. The Company shall not be required to segregate on its books or otherwise any amount to be used for the payment of benefits under the Plan.

SECTION 6

Other Employment

A Participant shall not be required to mitigate the amount of any payment or benefit provided for under the Plan by seeking other employment or otherwise nor shall the amount of any payment or benefit provided for under the Plan be reduced by any compensation earned by the Participant as a result of other employment.

SECTION 7

Miscellaneous

7.1.   Information to be Furnished by Participants. Each Participant must furnish to the Committee such documents, evidence, data or other information, as the Committee considers necessary or desirable for the purpose of administering the Plan. Benefits under the Plan for each Participant are provided on the condition that he furnish full, true and complete data, evidence or other information, and that he will promptly sign any document related to the Plan, requested by the Committee.

7.2. <u>Claims Review</u>. Any claim for benefits under the Plan or a Participant's Agreement by a Participant shall be made in writing and delivered to the Committee. If a Participant, or any beneficiary following the Participant's death (collectively, the "Claimant"), believes he has been denied any benefits or payments under the Plan or Agreement, either in total or in an amount less than the full benefit or payment to which the Claimant would normally be entitled, the Committee shall advise the Claimant in writing of the amount of the benefit, or payment, if any, and the specific reasons for the denial. The Committee shall also furnish the Claimant at that time with a written notice containing:

(a)   A specific reference to pertinent provisions of the Plan or the Participant's Agreement;

(b)   A description of any additional material or information necessary for the Claimant to perfect the claim if possible, and an explanation of why such material or information is needed; and

(c)   An explanation of the claim review procedure is set forth below. Within 60 days of receipt of the information described above, a Claimant shall, if further review is desired, file a written request for reconsideration with the Committee. So long as the Claimant's request for review is pending (including such 60-day period), Claimant or his duly authorized representative may review pertinent documents and may submit issues and comments in writing to the Committee. A final and binding decision shall be made by the Committee within 60 days of the filing by the Claimant of the request for reconsideration; provided, however, that if the Committee, in its discretion, feels that a hearing with the Claimant or his representative present is necessary or desirable, this period shall be extended an additional 60 days. The decision by the Committee shall be conveyed to the Claimant in writing and shall include specific reasons for the decision, written in a manner calculated to be understood by the Claimant, which specifically pertinent provisions of the Plan or the Participant's Agreement on which the decision is based. The Committee shall use ordinary care and diligence in the performance of its duties.

7.3. Evidence. Evidence required of anyone under the Plan may be by certificate, affidavit, document or other information, which the person relying thereon considers pertinent and reliable, and signed, made or presented by the proper party or parties.

7.4. Fees and Expenses. The Company shall pay all reasonable legal fees and related expenses (including the reasonable costs of experts, evidence and counsel), when and as incurred by a Participant, as a result of contesting or disputing any termination of employment of the Participant following a Change in Control whether or not such contest or dispute is resolved in the Participant's favor but only if the Participant was seeking in good faith to obtain or enforce any right or benefit provided by the Plan or the Participant's Agreement or by any other plan or arrangement maintained by the Employers under which the Participant is or may be entitled to receive benefits.

7.5. Action by Employer. Any action required of or permitted by the Company under the Plan shall be by resolution of its Board of Directors, by resolution of a duly authorized committee of its Board of Directors, or by a person or persons authorized by resolutions of its Board of Directors or such committee.

7.6. Controlling Laws. Except to the extent superseded by laws of the United States, the laws of California shall be controlling in all matters relating to the Plan.

7.7. Interests Not Transferable. The interests of persons entitled to benefits under the Plan are not subject to their debts or other obligations and, except as may be required by the tax withholding provisions of the Internal Revenue Code or any state's income tax act, or pursuant to an agreement between a Participant and the Employers, may not be voluntarily sold, transferred, alienated, assigned or encumbered.

7.8. <u>Mistake of Fact</u>. Any mistake of fact or misstatement of fact shall be corrected when it becomes known and proper adjustment made by reason thereof.

7.9. <u>Severability</u>. In the event any provision of the Plan or an Agreement shall be held to be illegal or invalid for any reason, such illegality or invalidity shall not affect the remaining parts of the Plan or Agreement, and the Plan or Agreement shall be construed and enforced as if such illegal or invalid provisions had never been contained in the Plan or Agreement.

7.10. <u>Withholding</u>. The Company will withhold from any amounts payable under the Plan all federal, state, city and local taxes as shall be legally required and any applicable insurance premiums, as well as any other amounts authorized or required by Company policy including, but not limited to, withholding for garnishments and judgments or other court orders.

7.11. <u>Effect on Other Plans or Agreements</u>. Payments or benefits provided to a Participant under any Company, deferred compensation, savings, retirement or other employee benefit plan are governed solely by the terms of such plan. Any obligations or duties of a Participant pursuant to any non-competition or other agreement with the Company shall not be affected by the receipt of benefits under this Plan.

SECTION 8

Amendment and Termination

8.1. <u>Amendment and Termination</u>. New Era reserves the right to amend the Plan at any time or to terminate the Plan at any time provided that no such amendment or termination of the Plan shall affect the provisions of any Participant's Agreement then in force under the Plan.

Agreement Under New Era Health ServicesCorporation Change in Control Plan

THIS AGREEMENT is made as of June ___, 2001 by and between NEW ERA HEALTH SYSTEM, a California non-profit corporation (the "New Era"), [Insert name of employer if Executive does not work for New Era] and _____ ("Executive") under the New Era Health System Change in Control Plan (the "Plan").

WHEREAS, New Era considers the maintenance of a vital management group to be essential to protecting and enhancing the best interests of New Era and its members and to that end New Era has established the Plan to provide benefits to certain management employees in the event their employment is terminated following a change in control of New Era, participation in which Plan is evidenced by an individual agreement between New Era and each participating employee; and

WHEREAS, Executive is employed by _____ ("Employer") and is a member of the management group of Employer and New Era has determined that to reinforce and encourage the continued attention and dedication of Executive to his duties free from distractions which could arise in anticipation of or subsequent to a Change in Control of New Era, it should extend participation in the Plan to Executive;

NOW, THEREFORE, in consideration of the mutual covenants contained herein, New Era and Executive agree that Executive shall become a Participant in the Plan subject to the following terms which form a part of the Plan with respect to Executive's participation therein.

1. <u>Term and Nature of Agreement</u>. This Agreement and Executive's participation in the Plan shall commence as of the date hereof and shall continue in effect until the earlier of (a) twenty-four (24) months after a Change in Control or (b) June 30, 2002. As of June 30, 2002 and each third June 30 occurring thereafter, this Agreement shall be automatically renewed for a term of three (3) years unless New Era gives written notice to Executive at least 90 days prior to the renewal date that this Agreement will not be extended. Notwithstanding the foregoing, if a Change in Control (as hereinafter defined) occurs during the last two (2) years of any term of this Agreement, the term of this Agreement and Executive's Plan participation shall automatically be extended for a period of twenty-four (24) months after the end of the month in which the Change in Control occurs. If Executive's employment with New Era terminates prior to a Change in Control, this Agreement and Executive's participation in the Plan shall automatically expire. Furthermore, Executive may terminate this Agreement and his participation in the Plan at any time by giving New Era 30 days' advance written notice. This Agreement which evidences Executive's participation in the Plan shall be construed and enforced under Executive Retirement Income Security Act of 1974, as amended ("ERISA") as an unfunded welfare benefit plan. The Plan and this Agreement shall be administered by the Executive Compensation Committee of the Board of Directors of New Era (the "Committee").

2. <u>Severance Benefits Following a Change in Control</u>. If Employee's employment with Employer is terminated upon or within thirty-six (36) months following a Change in Control, Executive shall be entitled to the following severance benefits (in addition to any nonseverance compensation and benefits provided for under any of Employer's employee benefit plans, policies and practices or under the terms of any other contracts, but in lieu of

any severance pay under any Employer employee benefit plan, policy and practice or under the terms of any other contract including any employment contract):

(a) If Executive's employment is terminated by reason of Executive's disability, retirement or death or by Executive other than for Good Reason, Employer shall pay Executive his full base salary through the Date of Termination at the rate in effect at the time of termination (or the date of death in the case of Executive's death), plus any bonus or incentive compensation award which, pursuant to the terms of any compensation or incentive plan, Executive is entitled to receive but which has not yet been paid. If any bonus or incentive compensation plan provides for an award upon the achievement of certain goals by the end of a fiscal year or other time period and the Date of Termination occurs prior to the end of such time period or fiscal year, no award shall be made.

(b) If Executive's employment is terminated for Cause, Employer shall pay Executive his full base salary through the Date of Termination at the rate in effect at the time Notice of Termination is given plus any bonus or incentive compensation award which, pursuant to the terms of any compensation or incentive plan, Executive is entitled to receive but which has not yet been paid. If any bonus or incentive compensation plan provides for an award upon the achievement of certain goals by the end of a fiscal year or other time period and the Date of Termination occurs prior to the end of such time period or fiscal year, no award shall be made.

(c) If Executive's employment is terminated by Employer other than for Cause or by Executive for Good Reason, then: Within five (5) days after the Date of Termination, Employer shall pay Executive his full base salary through the Date of Termination at the greater of the rate in effect at the time the Change in Control occurred or the rate in effect when the Notice of Termination was given plus all sums previously awarded but not yet paid to Executive, pursuant to Employer's Executive Compensation Program. If any bonus or incentive compensation plan provides for an award upon the achievement of certain goals by the end of a fiscal year or other time period and the Date of Termination occurs prior to the end of such time period or fiscal year, no award shall be made;

(i) Employer shall pay Executive a gross severance benefit equal to the product of _____ times the Executive's Annual Base Salary at the greater of the rate in effect at the time the Change in Control occurred or the rate in effect when Notice of Termination was given. The severance benefit shall be paid during the ensuing _____-month period in equal installments according to Employer's normal payroll schedule beginning with the first payroll period in which Executive's Date of Termination occurs. Executive's "Annual Base Salary" shall mean the yearly salary rate established from time to time by Employer as Executive's regular salary for the next succeeding twelve (12) month period, payable pursuant to Employer's payroll on a periodic basis;

(ii) Employer shall provide all medical and other benefits for the Severance Period (as defined below) as in effect immediately prior to the Change in Control, including, without limitation, the continued use of any Employer-owned automobile, which shall be returned to Employer at the end of the Severance Period; and

(iv) New Era shall pay the costs of a reasonable outplacement service until Executive is employed on a full time basis.

3.   Non-Solicitation. In consideration for the severance benefits called for under paragraph 2(c) above, Executive agrees that during the 24-month period following his Date of Termination (the "Severance Period"), Executive will not, without the prior written consent of New Era, alone or in association with others, solicit on behalf of Executive, or any Competing Business, any employee of New Era, or any of New Era Affiliates, for employment with a Competing Business.

"Competing Business" shall mean any person or persons or entity or entities engaged in any business or activity engaged in by the Company. Should Executive fail to comply with the restrictions contained in this Section 3, this Agreement shall immediately terminate and Executive shall forfeit any remaining unpaid benefits under this Agreement.

4.   Other Employment. Executive shall not be required to mitigate the amount of any payment or benefit provided for under this Agreement by seeking other employment or otherwise nor shall the amount of any payment or benefit provided for in this Agreement be reduced by any compensation earned by Executive as a result of other employment. Payment to Executive pursuant to this Agreement shall constitute the entire obligation of Employer for severance pay and full settlement of any claim for severance pay under law or in equity that Executive might otherwise assert against Employer or any of its employees, officers or directors on account of Executive's termination.

5.   Change in Control. For purposes of the Plan a "Change in Control" shall have occurred if: (a) any "Person" (as such term is used in Sections 13(d) and 14(d) of the Securities Exchange Act of 1934, as amended ("Exchange Act") other than New Era), becomes the "beneficial owner" (as such term is defined in rule 13d-3 under the Exchange Act), directly or indirectly, of memberships of New Era representing 20% or more of the combined voting power of New Era's then outstanding memberships;

(b) during any period of not more than 24 months, individuals who at the beginning of such period constitute the Board of Directors of New Era, and any new director (other than a director designated by a Person who has entered into an agreement with New Era to effect a transaction described in paragraph (a), (c), or (d) of this Section 5) whose election by the board or nomination for election by New Era's members was approved by a vote of at least two-thirds of the directors then still in office who either were directors at the beginning of the period or whose election or nomination for election was previously so approved, cease for any reason to constitute at least a majority thereof; (c) the Board of Directors of New Era approves a merger or consolidation of New Era or New Era Hospital Association (the "Association") with any other corporation, other than (i) a merger or consolidation which would result in the voting memberships of New Era outstanding immediately prior thereto continuing to represent (by being converted into voting memberships of the surviving entity) more than 60% of the combined voting power of the voting memberships of New Era or such surviving entity outstanding immediately after such merger or consolidation, or (ii) a merger or consolidation effected to implement a recapitalization of New Era (or similar transaction) in which no Person acquires more than 20% of the combined voting power of New Era's then outstanding memberships; or (d) the Board of Directors of New Era approves a plan of complete liquidation of New Era or the Association or an agreement for the sale or disposition by New Era or the Association of all or substantially all of its assets (or any transaction having a similar effect).

6.   Terminations for Cause and Good Reason. Executive will be considered to have been terminated for "Cause" if the termination is by reason of Executive willfully engaging in conduct demonstrably and materially injurious to Employer or tending to bring Employer into disrepute, Executive's commission of any illegal, unethical or dishonest act in connection with his

employment relationship or Executive's willful and continued failure for a significant period of time to perform Executive's duties after a demand for substantial performance has been delivered to Executive by the Board of Directors of Employer which demand specifically identifies the manner in which the Board believes that Executive has not substantially performed his duties. Executive's termination shall be considered to have been for "Good Reason" if Executive's termination is by reason of the occurrence of any of the following events within 24 months following a Change in Control without Executive's express written consent:

(a) any change in Executive's title, authorities, responsibilities (including reporting responsibilities) which, in Executive's reasonable judgment, represents an adverse change; the assignment to Executive of any duties or work responsibilities which, in his reasonable judgment, are inconsistent with such title, authorities or responsibilities; or any removal of Executive from, or failure to reappoint or reelect him to any of such positions, except if any such changes are because of disability, retirement or Cause;

(b) a reduction in or failure to pay any portion of Executive's Annual Base Salary as in effect on the date of the Change in Control or as the same may be increased from time to time thereafter;

(c) the failure by Employer to provide Executive with compensation and benefits (including, without limitation, incentive, bonus and other compensation plans and any vacation, medical, hospitalization, life insurance, dental or disability benefit plan), or cash compensation in lieu thereof, which are, in the aggregate, no less favorable than those provided by Employer to Executive immediately prior to the occurrence of the Change in Control;

(d) any breach by Employer of any provision of this Agreement; and

(e) the failure of Employer and New Era to obtain a satisfactory agreement from any successor or assign of Employer and New Era to assume and agree to perform this Agreement, as required in Section 8 of this Agreement.

Executive's continued employment after the expiration of 60 days from any action which would constitute Good Reason under paragraph 6(a) above shall constitute a waiver of rights with respect to such action constituting Good Reason under this Agreement.

7. Notice of Termination. Any purported termination of employment by Employer or by Executive shall be communicated by a written Notice of Termination to the other party which notice is given in accordance with Section 10 of this Agreement. No purported termination shall be effective without such a Notice of Termination. The Notice of Termination shall set forth in reasonable detail the facts and circumstances claimed to provide a basis for termination of Executive's employment and shall specify the Date of Termination. The "Date of Termination" shall mean the date specified in the Notice of Termination provided that in no case shall the date be less than thirty (30) days or more than sixty (60) days after the date the Notice of Termination is given.

8. Successors. New Era and Employer will require any successor or assign (whether direct or indirect, by purchase, merger, consolidation or otherwise) to all or substantially all of the business and/or assets of New Era and/or Employer to expressly assume and agree to perform this Agreement in the same manner and to the same extent New Era and Employer would be required to perform if no such succession or assignment had taken place. As used in this Agreement, "New Era" and "Employer" shall include any successor or assign to their business and/or assets which assumes and agrees to perform this Agreement by operation of law, or otherwise. This Agreement shall inure to the benefit of and be enforceable by Executive's personal and legal representatives, executors, administrators, successors, heirs, distributees, devisees and legatees. If Executive should die while any amounts would still be payable to him hereunder if he had continued to live, all such amounts, unless

otherwise provided herein, shall be paid in accordance with the terms of this Agreement to Executive's beneficiary and if there is no such beneficiary, to Executive's estate in a lump sum.

9.   Fees and Expenses. Employer shall pay all reasonable legal fees and related expenses (including the reasonable costs of experts, evidence and counsel), when and as incurred by Executive, as a result of contesting or disputing any termination of employment of Executive following a Change in Control whether or not such contest or dispute is resolved in Executive's favor but only if Executive was seeking in good faith to obtain or enforce any right or benefit provided by this Agreement or by any other plan or arrangement maintained by New Era or Employer under which Executive is or may be entitled to receive benefits.

10.   Notice. Any notice or other communication provided for or required by this Agreement shall be in writing and shall be deemed to have been duly given when personally delivered or sent by certified mail, return receipt requested, postage prepaid, addressed to the respective addresses last given by each party to the other or to such other address as either party may have furnished to the other in writing.

11.   Modifications, Waivers and Survival of Obligations. No provision of this Agreement may be modified, waived or discharged unless such modification, waiver or discharge is agreed to in writing and signed by Executive, Employer and New Era. A waiver of any condition or provision of this Agreement shall be limited to the terms and conditions of such waiver and shall be not be construed as a waiver of any similar or dissimilar provisions or condition at any time. The obligations of New Era and Employer under Section 2 shall survive the expiration of the term of this Agreement.

12.   Claims Procedure. Any claim for benefits under this Agreement by Executive shall be made in writing pursuant to the claims procedure stated in the Plan.

13. Governing Law. The laws of California shall be controlling in all matters relating to this Agreement and the Plan to the extent not preempted by ERISA.

14. Severability. The provisions of this Agreement shall be deemed severable and the invalidity or unenforceability of any provision shall not affect the validity or enforceability of the other provisions hereof.

15. Entire Agreement. This Agreement constitutes the entire agreement between the parties hereto and supersedes all prior agreements, understandings and arrangements, oral or written, between the parties hereto with respect to the subject matter hereof.

16. Action by New Era or Employer. Any action required of or permitted by New Era or Employer under this Agreement shall be by resolution of its applicable Board of Directors, by resolution of a duly authorized committee of the applicable Board of Directors, or by a person or persons authorized by resolutions of the applicable Board of Directors or such committee.

17. Counterparts. This Agreement may be executed in several counterparts, each of which shall be deemed to be an original but all of which together will constitute one and the same instrument.

18. Non-Exclusivity of Rights. Nothing in this Agreement shall prevent or limit Executive's continuing or future participation in any benefit, bonus, incentive or other plan or program provided by New Era or Employer and for which Executive may qualify, nor shall anything herein limit or reduce such rights as Executive may have under any other agreements with New Era or Employer. Amounts which are vested benefits or which Executive is otherwise entitled to receive under any plan or program of New Era or Employer shall be payable in accordance with such plan or program, except as explicitly modified by this Agreement.

NEW ERA HEALTH SYSTEM
By: _____
Title:

_____
Employee
[Insert Employer's name if New Era
is not Employer]
By: _____
Title

Note: "New Era Health Systems" is a fictional entity. Any resemblance to an actual entity is purely coincidental.

CHAPTER 7

Recruiting Healthcare Executives

Jack Schlosser

WHEN IT COMES to lines of business, the field of professional search consulting is a relative newcomer. The first institutionalized healthcare systems, in the form of hospitals, appeared on the scene more than a millennium ago; by contrast, the first businesses specializing in recruiting professional managers emerged only in the aftermath of World War II.

Over the past half century, the executive search industry has grown from a handful of firms conducting dozens of searches to scores of firms conducting thousands of searches. According to the Association of Executive Search Consultants (AESC) web site (www.aesc.org), an international trade group based in New York and Brussels, every year some 10,000 searches take place around the world.

The growth of the AESC itself shows how far the industry has come. Founded as a small organization in 1959, today it represents 160 leading search firms. These firms collectively boast some 700 offices and more than 3,500 search consultants around the globe— all of them working on retainers. Moreover, the AESC represents only a fraction of the firms in existence. The growth of the search industry, paralleling that of industry in general, has developed to the point that today literally thousands of companies offer some type of workforce recruiting services. Some of these receive a retainer from the hiring company, like AESC members, but many also work for companies on a contingency, or accept payment from individuals seeking employment. Counting all of these matchmakers, the field of search consultants is broad indeed.

AN OVERVIEW OF EXECUTIVE RECRUITING IN HEALTHCARE

The rise of the executive search industry has changed the nature of human resource development in healthcare. Most hospitals and health systems today at least consider using a search firm to help recruit at the CEO level, and most senior healthcare executives have regular contact with executive recruiters as either clients or candidates.

Search firms are categorized by the way they are compensated. One key distinction is whether a firm is working for the company that is hiring, or for the individual who seeks to be hired. Looking only at search firms paid by companies, another distinction is whether the company is paid on a retainer basis or by contingency. Contingency companies are paid only if the candidates they present to a client are actually hired by the client. Such firms typically work below the executive level. Retainer firms such as Spencer Stuart, similar in fee structure to law firms, are compensated for providing more comprehensive services in defining and meeting the client's needs. These firms seek executive leadership at the highest levels of the organization—from senior management to boards of directors.

The healthcare industry is a relatively heavy user of executive search services—and has been since the establishment of federal health programs in nations around the world. In the United States, the trend began with the advent of Medicare and Medicaid programs in the mid-1960s. Federal healthcare programs, as well as the dollars and expectations that came with them, quickly led to the development of healthcare management as a profession. The old ways of managing became inadequate to deal with the massive changes occurring. Healthcare became an industry—an industry that needed leaders. As hospital administration evolved into a professional management discipline, demand for the services of executive search consultants grew accordingly.

Medicare and Medicaid generated both new sources of revenues and new costs. The federal government paid healthcare providers for the services they administered to Medicare and Medicaid beneficiaries. At the same time, the Medicare and Medicaid programs mandated a number of organizational changes. Many provider organizations, with some help from the federal government, have devoted some of their revenue stream to train their managers to cope with these changes.

HEALTHCARE LEADERSHIP

Healthcare management is rightfully known as one of most demanding leadership challenges, and the major industry trends of the past three decades have only escalated the importance of attracting and retaining top management in this field. The revolutionary impact of federal healthcare programs is only one of the changes that the healthcare field has sustained in this generation. Two other trends deserve at least brief mention—consolidation and fragmentation. Healthcare institutions are combining with one another at a rapid rate, both through mergers of equals and through "roll-ups" of previously independent healthcare firms (i.e., home healthcare firms) thus causing greater concentration of market share in fewer leading organizations. At the same time, the field is becoming more fragmentary with the rapid emergence of the first and second generations of entrepreneurial startups—a phenomenon that is being exponentially increased by the recent major advances in biotechnology and genomics.

As a result of all these trends, the healthcare industry is especially in need of visionary leadership capable of developing innovative responses to continuing competitive and financial challenges.

The 21st Century Health Care Leader, a compendium of leading thought in the field, contains a number of valuable insights on leadership of the modern healthcare organization. In one chapter, Emory University faculty members John D. Henry, Sr. and Roderick W. Gilkey observe, "We are living in a time when a new form of leadership—leadership as the ability to inspire, empower and exert broad influence—supplants leadership as the exercise of centralized power and control" (Henry and Gilkey 1999). How can healthcare organizations attract a leader of this caliber, one capable of building a team of senior executives who can move an organization through today's complex environment to continuing growth and profitability? This is a difficult and very often expensive task, but one well worth the price tag if it is done right.

The extremes of large consolidated organizations versus newly formed cutting-edge health sciences firms present a unique challenge to the executive recruiter who is charged with finding seasoned leaders. Some major healthcare systems have grown so large that it is extremely difficult to find candidates experienced at heading such huge organizations, and the world of startups is also largely uncharted in terms of leadership. With new ground being broken organizationally in both areas, and with both demanding results-oriented executives, healthcare boards and their advisors are forced to look for new paradigms of talent. A search for "parallel experience" is a good start, but leaders and their advisors must also look to new skill sets and competencies in recruiting for these types of organizations.

Meanwhile, both market dynamics and demographics are contributing to a smaller pool of talent as the vast Baby Boom generation reaches retirement age and is succeeded by less populous generations of workers. But it should also be noted that the extremes of low supply and high demand apply most intensely at the top of the pool. Only a very small group of senior executives—the top 5 to 10 percent of the workforce—moves in this arena.

Overall workforce shortages are separate from, and much milder than, this highly publicized war for top talent—one in which the competition to attract a star may take compensation elements to new and, at times, seemingly inappropriate highs. In such cases, the search professional can be a voice of reason, supplying data and options that will keep negotiations at a realistic level without depriving the client of superlative talent.

HOW THE SEARCH PROCESS WORKS

A good search consultant can help a client organization recruit senior executives in a variety of ways—from identifying high-potential candidates to helping fine-tune a compensation package.

Companies in need of a search consultant should contact several firms and compare their services. No reputable search firm will resent such a "contest." Indeed, winning the assignment is the first step for any search firm. Once the client is engaged, basic steps of the executive search process are followed:

- *Starting the search.* In this phase, the client, consultant, and associate jointly agree on the basic parameters of the search. The consultant and the client hold a briefing meeting to analyze and establish the required competencies, understand key relationships, define the required experience, and identify other factors needed to attract the ideal candidate. From this briefing, a written position specification is prepared, outlining the position, key relationships, major responsibilities, ideal experience, ideal personal profile, and key competencies required for the position.
- *Identifying prospects.* In this stage, one of the most intensive of the search, the consulting firm expands research efforts and makes calls to targeted sources and prospects to identify and prequalify high-quality potential candidates for the position.

- *Developing candidates.* At this point, the consultant interviews and evaluates the best prospects identified in the previous phase and begins educating the most promising candidates about the opportunity.
- *Presenting candidates.* The consultant presents written and verbal evaluations of the best candidates to the client, and the client and consultant agree on how candidates should be interviewed by the client organization.
- *Preparing for the close.* In this phase, the consultant plays a crucial role in facilitating the negotiations between client and finalist to speed progress toward a successful placement. Referencing of the top candidates is a very important step in the process. During this phase, the consultant gathers insights and comments about the top candidates from people qualified to evaluate their abilities based on the competencies required for the position.
- *Closing placement.* The organization makes a formal offer to the candidate, and the candidate accepts the offer, negotiates a different offer, or (in rare cases) rejects the offer. The step-by-step approach outlined above, if practiced correctly, can bring with it an element of trust that proves beneficial at "crunch time" when the searching organization and its consultant are trying to convince the candidate to sign on.
- *Post-search follow-up.* As the candidate approaches and then assumes the new responsibilities, the consultant follows up periodically with both the client and the candidate to encourage a smooth transition into the company and informs/thanks other candidates, prospects, and sources who have been helpful during the search.

NEGOTIATING THE COMPENSATION PACKAGE

Having a consultant manage this entire process allows the board search committee (in the case of a CEO search) or executive team to focus on the essence of the search: the candidate's competencies and fit with the organization. Working from databases, consultants are able to gather precise information not only about the candidates but also about their environments, including norms, standards, and new developments in compensation.

The value of a search consultant in the process of negotiating a compensation package is basically that of a credible third party and objective facilitator for each side. The search consultant is immersed in the marketplace and in constant contact with people and organizations in the healthcare industry. Thus, one of the benefits he or she brings to the table is an intimate knowledge of the human capital side of healthcare.

Very often, for example, search consultants possess comparative compensation data such as industry or market norms for comparable positions at competing organizations, as well as informed estimates of the current compensation levels of candidates. This empirical market information can complement detailed information provided by compensation consultants. Working together, the search consultant and compensation consultant position the search for a successful conclusion by knowing and sharing the realities of the marketplace.

Without careful communication and management of expectations, a recruit who comes with a high price tag is often unable to live up to the expectations of the board, expectations that may or may not be realistic or achievable. The recruiting period is the time to hammer out these criteria—not the first six months on the job. A good search consultant is adept at leading this process, and works to ensure a smooth transition for the successful placement.

One of the trickiest aspects of constructing the compensation package is achieving the right balance between offering too much, so that the candidate starts out in a defensive position in justifying his or her value to the organization, versus offering too little and making the organization vulnerable to poaching by competitors because of inadequate investment in the candidate up front.

During negotiations, the number of key players tends to contract. In healthcare, as in other industries, the search begins with the involvement of a full search committee, but as the time for negotiation with a lead candidate approaches, the team generally narrows to just a few key parties.

The negotiating team ideally consists of only a handful of people: typically, the chair of the search committee, the chair of the board's compensation committee, the compensation consultant who helps design the compensation program, and the search consultant. A small group ensures less confusion and less opportunity for inconsistencies and second-guessing. Once this group has assembled the package, it typically goes back to the board for approval before the organization extends a final offer.

Thus, from the time a lead candidate is identified, and throughout the process of waiting for the reference checks, the search consultant is deeply involved in the negotiating process—not only with the "starring" candidate but also "behind the scenes." Several fallback candidates are usually chosen as well, and the search consultant maintains contact with these other candidates in the event the lead candidate falls through. The consultant must strike a difficult balance between keeping the other candidates interested and not misleading them with hopes that may prove false if the current negotiations are successful.

During the pay negotiation stage, the search consultant's relationship-building really benefits the client; if the search firm has done its job well, it will be in a position of strong credibility and trust with all the players. The search consultant acts as a "shuttle diplomat" during this period, touching base with all the parties and keeping everything in motion. These negotiations may take days, or even weeks.

While the search consultant facilitates the offer—and at the client's request may even float a draft offer—the actual final offer should come from the client. If the search consultant has been an effective liaison, there should be few, if any, surprises by the time the offer is extended.

SEARCH ETHICS

Being an honest broker among all the parties is of supreme importance for the search consultant. Yet the work of an honest broker does not come automatically; it requires a concerted effort by all parties involved in the search process.

The pervasiveness of executive recruiting has given rise to the potential for conflicts of interest. As mentioned at the outset of this chapter, most healthcare executives have contact with executive recruiters either as clients or as candidates. In some cases, healthcare executives might find themselves in a position to be both a client and a candidate—clearly a conflict of interest. For this reason and similar reasons, professionals in the field have devised guidelines for ethical and professional conduct.

From day one, Spencer Stuart has operated according to the unique vision of its founder: that executive search is a consultative, relationship-based business centered around the long-term success of clients. This groundbreaking approach has led to policies and practices that are now firm—and industry—standards.

One widely followed set of ethical and professional standards for executive search comes from the AESC. Since its founding over 40 years ago, the AESC has sought to promote high standards of professionalism among its members. In furtherance of this aim, AESC adopted a *Code of Ethics* in 1977 (*Code*), and a set of *Professional Practice Guidelines* in 1984 (*Guidelines*). In 1996, the AESC revised and updated both the *Code* and the *Guidelines* to reflect important developments in the profession and the business environment.

The AESC's updated *Code* asserts the fundamental principles that should guide executive search consultants in their work, as seen in Figure 7.1. The *Guidelines* represent the AESC members' view of the "best practices" for executive search consultants (see Appendix 7A at the end of this chapter). The AESC has stated that it may amend its *Guidelines* "as the profession evolves and adapts to developments in business practices, technology, and law" (AESC 1996).

Figure 7.1: AESC *Code of Ethics*

The Association of Executive Search Consultants, Inc. (AESC) is a world-wide association of retained executive search consulting firms. In order to perform their duties responsibly, AESC member firms are guided by the following ethical principles

Professionalism: conduct their activities in a manner that reflects favorably on the profession.

Integrity: conduct their business activities with integrity and avoid conduct that is deceptive or misleading.

Competence: perform all search consulting assignments competently, and with an appropriate degree of knowledge, thoroughness, and urgency.

Objectivity: exercise objective and impartial judgment in each search consulting assignment, giving due consideration to all relevant facts.

Accuracy: strive to be accurate in all communications with clients and candidates and encourage them to exchange relevant and accurate information.

Conflicts of Interest: avoid, or resolve through disclosure and waiver, conflicts of interest.

Confidentiality: respect confidential information entrusted to them by clients and candidates.

Loyalty: serve their clients loyally and protect client interests when performing assignments.

Equal Opportunity: support equal opportunity in employment and objectively evaluate all qualified candidates.

Public Interest: conduct their activities with respect for the public interest.

Source: Association of Executive Search Consultants. 1996. Code of Ethics. New York: AESC. [Online information; retrieved 2/5/02]. http://www.aesc.org/ethics.html.

SIDE ISSUES THAT CAN MAKE OR BREAK DEAL

Because of the early and continuing communications with candidates, search consultants are also in a position to help clients address indirect compensation issues such as spousal employment, school issues involving children, and real estate issues. While these may seem to be peripheral, any one of these issues can potentially cause a carefully constructed deal to collapse. Again, candidates often feel more comfortable communicating their concerns about these areas to a neutral but trustworthy third party: the search consultant. Getting the concerns on the table is the first essential step to finding solutions.

A related issue in which search professionals play a role is that of "selling" the community where the position is located. Consultants can provide cost-of-living comparisons and information that plays a key role in determining compensation. If an organization is trying to move a candidate from Fargo, North Dakota, to Irvine, California, for example, significant cost-of-living issues exist. In such a case it is important to determine, fairly early in the process, whether it is realistic, or even possible, for a candidate to make this move. The search consultant can help create the dialogue that leads to a prompt resolution of these issues. Again, however, the consultant works in concert with other professionals, in this case relocation consultants, who are the real experts in the specific details of the relocation itself.

Here, as in the post-offer process, the ultimate value of the search consultant is that he or she has built up a trusting and credible relationship with all the parties involved and can help move the process forward neutrally and swiftly toward an amiable conclusion.

CONCLUSION

"Newcomer" or not, executive search is here to stay—especially in critically important fields such as healthcare. Organizations dedicated to public health today need to identify and hire the right leaders—individuals with the special skills and qualities needed to help them serve to the fullest. Executive recruiters, more than ever before, can help organizations to obtain that talent.

REFERENCES

Association of Executive Search Consultants (AESC). 1996. *Code of Ethics.* New York: AESC. [Online information; retrieved 2/5/02]. http://www.aesc.org/ethics.html.

Association of Executive Search Consultants (AESC). 1996. *Professional Practice Guidelines.* New York: AESC. [Online information; retrieved 2/5/02]. http://www.aesc.org/practice.html.

Henry, J. D., Sr., and R. W. Gilkey. 1999. "Growing Effective Leadership in New Organizations." In *The 21st Century Health Care Leader,* edited by R. W. Gilkey, San Francisco: Jossey-Bass.

The Association of Executive Search Consultants Professional Practice Guidelines

RELATIONSHIPS BETWEEN AESC MEMBERS AND THEIR CLIENTS

AESC members are partners with their clients in a consultative process aimed at selecting organizational leaders. The success of these partnerships depends on excellence in client service. The following guidelines describe the processes and professional practices that contribute to outstanding client service.

ACCEPTING CLIENT ASSIGNMENTS

Outstanding client service begins with a full understanding of the client organization, its business needs and the position to be filled. An AESC member should:

Accept only those assignments that a member is qualified to undertake on the basis of the member's knowledge of the client's needs and the member's ability to perform the specific assignment.

Accept only those assignments that will not adversely affect the member's objectivity, loyalty, and integrity.

Disclose to present and prospective clients information known to the member about relationships, circumstances or interests that might create actual or potential conflicts of interest, and accept potential assignments only if all affected parties have expressly agreed to waive any conflict.

Disclose to present and prospective clients limitations arising through service to other clients that may affect the member's ability to perform the search assignment.

Base acceptances on an understanding that, among other things, defines the scope and character of the services to be provided; the identity of the client organization; the period, if any, during which the member will not recruit from the defined client organization; and the fees and expenses to be charged for the services rendered.

Discuss with the client when advertising is required by law or is a recommended strategy for the particular search assignment.

PERFORMING CLIENT ASSIGNMENTS

Members should serve their clients with integrity and objectivity, making every effort to conduct search consulting activities on the basis of impartial consideration of relevant facts. Specifically, an AESC member should:

Conduct an appropriate search for qualified candidates.

Advise the client promptly, and offer alternative courses of action if it becomes apparent that no qualified candidates can be presented, or that the length of the search will differ considerably from that originally specified.

Present information about the client, the position, and the candidate honestly and factually, and include reservations that are pertinent and important to an assignment.

Withdraw from the assignment if a member determines that a client has characterized its organization falsely or misled candidates, provided the situation is not rectified.

Thoroughly evaluate potential candidates, including: in-depth interviews in person or by video conferencing, verification of credentials, and careful assessment of the candidate's strengths and weaknesses, before presenting candidates for client interviews.

Complete thorough reference checks and transmit these references to the client.

Advise the client if advertising becomes necessary.

Avoid the voluntary presentation of resumes in the absence of an existing client relationship.

PRESERVING THE CONFIDENTIALITY OF CLIENT INFORMATION

AESC members should use their best efforts to protect confidential information concerning their clients. Specifically, a member should:

Use such confidential information received from clients only for purposes of conducting the assignment.

Disclose such confidential client information only to those individuals within the firm or to potential candidates who have a need to know the information.

Not use such confidential information for personal gain, nor provide inside information to third parties for their personal gain.

AVOIDING CONFLICTS OF INTEREST

AESC members should protect their integrity, objectivity, and loyalty by avoiding conflicts of interest with their clients. For example, a member should:

Refuse or withdraw from an assignment upon learning of conditions that impair the member's ability to perform services properly, including conflicts of interest that may arise during the assignment (unless all affected parties expressly agree to waive the conflict).

Inform clients of business or personal relationships with candidates that might affect or appear to affect the member's objectivity in conducting the assignment.

Not accept payment for assisting an individual in securing employment.

Avoid knowingly presenting simultaneously, without disclosure to clients, the same candidate to more than one client.

RELATIONSHIPS BETWEEN AESC MEMBERS AND CANDIDATES

Although a member's primary relationship is with the client, member firms seek also to establish professional relationships with candidates. These relationships should be characterized by honesty, objectivity, accuracy, and respect for confidentiality. In building such relationships, a member should:

Provide candidates with relevant and accurate information about the client organization and the position.

Present to clients accurate and relevant information about candidates, and otherwise maintain the confidentiality of information provided by prospective and actual candidates.

Encourage candidates to provide accurate information about their qualifications. Upon learning that a candidate has misled the client or member regarding his or her qualifications, the member should reject the candidate, unless the client, candidate and member agree that the candidacy should continue following disclosure of the facts.

Advise prospects and candidates of the status and disposition of their candidacies in a timely fashion.

Consider whether an individual's permission is needed before sharing his or her background information with a client and secure permission as necessary (permission should always be obtained if an executive's "resume" is submitted).

Advise candidates of any limitations on a member firm's ability to advance them as candidates in future searches.

RELATIONSHIPS BETWEEN AESC MEMBERS AND THEIR CONTRACTORS

AESC members sometimes rely on contractors and subcontractors to assist in the search process.

A member should:

Avoid contractors and subcontractors whose practices are inconsistent with the standards of professionalism expected of AESC members.

Encourage its contractors and subcontractors to adhere to the *Code of Ethics* and *Professional Practice Guidelines*.

RELATIONSHIPS BETWEEN AESC MEMBERS AND THE PUBLIC

AESC members should recognize the importance of public trust and confidence in their profession and seek to serve their clients in a manner consistent with the public interest.

Therefore, a member should:

Observe the principles of equal opportunity in employment and avoid unlawful discrimination against qualified candidates.

Promote and advertise member firm services in a professional and accurate manner.

Conduct relations with the media so as to reflect favorably upon the AESC, clients, and the executive search consulting profession.

Source: Association of Executive Search Consultants. 1996. *Professional Practice Guidelines*. New York: AESC. [Online information; retrieved 2/5/02]. http://www.aesc.org/practice.html.

CHAPTER 8

Physician Compensation

Charles A. Peck

ONE OF THE most important goals for any healthcare organization today is to align physician pay with institutional mission and vision. The old fee-for-service days, in which doctors were paid for each service they rendered, are waning. In their place is a complex reimbursement system that uses mixed methods for determining fees, which are often limited or "capitated" according to set formulas. As a result, institutions and physicians alike need to find new ways to ensure that physicians receive compensation commensurate with the value of their service.

The ideal compensation plan should move beyond traditional methods of measuring physician activity, such as panel size, number of encounters, or cost per visit. Instead, the plan should reward physicians for the value and quality of their work. Appropriate incentives for increasing this value and quality should also be included. The challenge, of course, is to balance that incentive-based compensation with efficiency, fiscal responsibility, and the provision of quality care—all in a mixed-fee, capitated payment environment. This combination is not easy to achieve. Indeed, if mismanaged, it can lead to a kind of operational schizophrenia, in which one hand is constantly undoing the good done by the other.

This clash of purposes has defeated many healthcare organizations, but it need not defeat yours. Quality care and reasonable cost can coexist, even in the most operationally schizophrenic environment. The key is for institutions to influence clinician behavior that is fiscally responsible yet medically appropriate through use of a suitable compensation formula. "Suitable" will be defined here as a formula that is ethical, fair, and flexible, while enhancing medical management and preventing illness.

Suitable physician compensation:

- Meets ethical standards for the level and nature of pay in healthcare.
- Compensates physicians fairly.
- Can flexibly suit the needs of institutions and physicians.
- Serves the needs of medical management.
- Rewards prevention of illness.

Using this definition for suitable compensation, one might well argue that setting suitable compensation for physicians is the single most important responsibility of any healthcare institution that engages physician services. Of course, meeting this definition requires that organizations understand certain key issues and principles. The purpose of this chapter is to discuss these issues and principles in the context of a healthcare organization that employs or contracts with physicians. Such organizations might include independent hospitals, affiliated hospital systems, or physician partnerships/joint ventures such as physician hospital organizations (PHO), a management services organization (MSO), or an independent physician association (IPA).

MEDICAL MANAGEMENT STRATEGY

First and foremost, the design of physician pay should align with the medical management strategy of the organization. This can occur if pay is designed holistically—with a design for total pay. The opportunity to redesign a physician compensation plan presents a wonderful chance to strengthen group culture. In particular, it can orient physicians towards corporate success by redefining important parameters of medical management, including the balance of quality care and revenue management.

Medical management is the process whereby an organization delivers clinical care services and measures clinical care results in a high-quality, cost-effective manner that achieves both patient and physician satisfaction. The key elements of a medical management strategy include:

- A provider compensation program that offers financial incentives for physicians while at the same time requiring them to share financial risks.
- A comprehensive health management program that includes both inpatient and outpatient care.
- An information system that can integrate claim data and clinical results, providing timely and comprehensive data that can help physicians measure quality, outcomes, and efficiency.
- A method to determine and measure "utilization appropriateness," that is fair and based upon the continuum of care required by the patient. In the end, an integration of all the healthcare services required by a patient will be more cost-effective than continued emphasis on episodes of acute care only.
- Education and involvement of key constituents.

To summarize, a compensation plan must be integrated with medical management to allow definition, monitoring, measurement, and improvement of quality and the lowering of practice costs. This said, let us now explore the components of an effective compensation design.

PAY PERCEPTION VERSUS REALITY

Any stated plan for physician pay should look as fair and reasonable as it is—no more, no less. Very often, there is a gap between perception and reality in this respect. For example, stakeholders may think the pay awarded to physicians is overly generous, when it fact it is based on a reasonable formula. Conversely, physicians may be dissatisfied with a pay plan that is in fact quite generous, simply because they do not understand how it will work.

It may seem simple to align perception and reality, but it is in fact quite difficult, given the complexity of physician pay today. Market dynamics, fee schedules, expense profiles, the mix of payers (that is customers paying for the healthcare, often employers), patient volume, referrals, managed care contracts, and third party payment schedules for different specialties—these are just a few of the variables that must be included in any formula. To the uninitiated, physician compensation can appear to be pure "Greek"—literally. Consider the many mathematical symbols (often expressed in Greek letters) appearing in the compensation plan model proposed by M. Gaynor and P. Gertler (1995) in their article on physician pay:

$$y_1 = \alpha P q_1 + (1/n)(1 - \alpha)P\sum_{j=1}^{n}q_1 - (1/n)FC - (1/n)WH$$

This article shows the oxymoron in the phrase "simple compensation plan." Another complicating factor is the highly personal nature of medical care, which adds a subjective element to its value—and evaluation.

The key to making a plan clear (thus aligning perception and reality) is to articulate exactly how the plan complements and fosters the mission and vision of the organization, as well as the organization's corporate culture and financial goals. Indeed, all these ideas must be clearly articulated to the satisfaction of all stakeholders involved, and consensus reached before plan design even begins.

For their part, physicians must understand clearly the premise under which they are being paid. For example, all parties involved need to understand the impact of referrals. A high level of specialty referral may cause a decrease in budgets for primary care. If this happens, the organization must make it clear that the budgeting "pie" is not being divided differently; it is shrinking. In this case, it will be important to increase communication and financial accountability between primary care doctors and specialists, to amend some of the traditional problems that can arise between these groups of physicians.

The "gold standard" for any compensation plan is to make it simple enough to explain to a physician's spouse or family member, and flexible enough to reward physicians for positive health outcomes. Clearly, it will be easier to meet this standard if the physician has helped define the basic parameters of the plan in the first place. This sense of ownership becomes critically important when shaping the plan for a multispecialty practice, where earning potentials may vary drastically between physicians. Physicians need to be involved in forming a plan for expense allocation, setting a value on internal referrals, and balancing department profitability and individual compensation. There are no shortcuts. Any approach that does not include the involvement and agreement of all physicians will doom even the most intricate actuarial and accounting gymnastics to a quick and undignified end.

PHYSICIAN PAY: FIVE KEY QUESTIONS TO ASK

By their very choice of profession, physicians tend to have a strong sense of propriety. Few if any are practicing medicine because they seek personal wealth. For this reason, some observers have suggested that physicians do not (or in any event should not) respond to economic incentives. However, the fact is that financial incentives can drive behavior. How healthcare providers are paid helps to determine the quality of care and outcomes that their patients realize. Research has shown a direct correlation between the level of quality delivered and the cost associated with that quality—the best way to lower cost is to improve quality. Apt incentives motivate physicians to effectively manage both care and costs.

Organizations that pay physicians based on straight salary increase their chances of failure, while organizations that align physician compensation packages with an effective and comprehensive health management system increase their chances of success. This has been shown through both negative and positive examples—some of them quite spectacular.[1]

Consequently, in revising a physician compensation plan, begin with these key questions:

1. Is the compensation plan motivating the right behaviors?
2. Are incentives properly driving high-quality patient outcomes?
3. Do the physicians understand the plan and how it may require practice adjustments?
4. Does the plan recognize and reward nonfinancial as well as financial outcomes (e.g., hard work, appropriate utilization, patient satisfaction, and service to the group)?
5. Are the providers satisfied and active supporters of the plan?

A key factor in innovative compensation design is the medical loss ratio (the percentage of every dollar spent on direct patient care). This ratio should be 78 to 80 percent. To ensure this result, a sufficient amount of each premium dollar must go to the provision of medical care. Some organizations achieve a percentage as high as 86 percent.

Early in the design phase of medical management strategy, the provider organization should negotiate with payers to get them to assume a greater share of the financial risk involved in operating the organization. As the group becomes more sophisticated and proficient in managing care and costs, it could conceivably take on even more risk and thus enhance reward potential.

EXAMPLES OF INCENTIVE PROGRAMS

To survive in today's competitive marketplace, plans need to integrate more than one payment mechanism. Capitation in and of itself is merely a payment imposed by a third-party payer. Therefore, even in organizations that are not yet heavily capitated, incentive-based mechanisms can be used to motivate physicians to change behaviors and actively focus on quality improvement and cost reduction. With this in mind, let us review several incentive options that can complement the fee-for-service component of the overall package.

- *Hard capitation.* This is the classic fixed payment-per-patient given to the provider. This system prevents churning—the unnecessary overutilization of patient visits. The hard capitation system typically means that the physician will provide few services, which in turn can bring more financial benefit to the physician because of lower utilization of resources and time. However this system tends to encourage suboptimal patient care, because the incentive is to do less. One way to offset this problem is to create a bonus pool that incentivizes quality care outcomes. Physicians who meet specific quality standards can obtain higher reimbursement. This does not always offset the problem completely, however, so many organizations have abandoned the hard capitation approach.
- *Contact compensation.* In this approach, specialty specific budgets are calculated based on historical benchmark and regional benchmark utilization, allocated for a specified period amount of time. The physicians themselves make the payment decisions from that capitated pool. A referral for specialist "contact" with the patient triggers a predetermined payment to cover costs of care. It is then left up to the specialist to determine the type of care that will be delivered, and any money left over will be paid to the provider as a bonus.

- *Shadow compensation.* Like the "contact compensation" approach, this one allocates budgets by specialty. However, the providers within each pool are actually paid on a fee-for-service basis until they hit the budgeted amount. Once this level of utilization is achieved, contact capitation begins. If physician groups have appropriate utilization protocols and never overutilize (that is, never overuse healthcare resources), they continue being reimbursed on a fee-for-service basis. Any money left in their budget is reallocated to them as a bonus.

- *Physician gainsharing.* The sharing of gain among physicians is another program that seemed to hold much promise for increasing quality and decreasing costs within a hospital physician practice. However, there are several real challenges to the implementation of a viable gainsharing partnership. Because of the dynamic nature of medical practice, it is not always easy to determine the contribution each physician makes to income, while ascertaining the costs each physician incurs.

PHYSICIAN GAINSHARING LANDMINES

In physician gainsharing, physicians and hospital executives form management redesign committees to generate cost savings by introducing new treatments and protocols. If these directives lead to lower costs of care, then the savings are shared between the physicians and the hospital. This type of program can be extremely effective in improving quality and decreasing costs, and physicians have been quite receptive to the concept.

Unfortunately, however, in a Special Advisory Bulletin dated July 8, 1999, the Office of the Inspector General (OIG) in the U.S. Health and Human Services declared hospital-physician gainsharing arrangements illegal for Medicare and Medicaid providers, surprising many in the healthcare industry. The bulletin focused on Section 1128A(b)(1) and (2) of the Social Security Act (42 U.S.C.

§ 1320a-7a(b) (1) and (2)), regulating hospital-sponsored physician incentive plans. The OIG interpreted this existing law as banning any hospital from knowingly making a payment, directly or indirectly, to a physician as an inducement to reduce or limit services to Medicare or Medicaid patients under the physician's direct care.

Among other provisions, the law prohibits "any hospital or critical access hospital from knowingly making a payment directly or indirectly to a physician as an inducement to reduce or limit services to Medicare or Medicaid beneficiaries under the physician's care" (OIG 1999). The only exceptions are risk-based Medicare managed care programs that have physician incentive programs in accordance with the relevant provisions of the Omnibus Budget Reconciliation Act of 1990 and subsequent (1992) federal rules.

Although many attorneys believe that the OIG's position is not a correct interpretation of the good law and could be challenged, no hospital or health system is willing to risk its Medicare accreditation to mount such a challenge. The OIG has said that legislation would be required to overturn the law. Given that no bills have been recently introduced to address this issue, hospitals must walk a fine line to avoid violating the law and paying the $2,000 per patient fine it exacts for such violations.

The U.S. General Accounting Office (GAO) in Washington, DC issued an often-cited report on the subject of physician incentive payments (GAO 1986). The report suggested that hospitals wanting to reduce the risk of compliance problems should:

- Base any payments to physicians an aggregated savings by groups of doctors.
- Consider physician performance over an extended period of time.
- Base payments on results with a large universe of patients rather than with individuals.
- Have strong utilization review and quality improvement protocols in place.

Despite any opinion on OIG's position on physician gainsharing, these four principles are actually very good management practices.

Another practice—and one that is consistent with the four suggestions above—is to have the hospitals enter into personal service contracts with physicians. In these contracts, physicians can be paid a fixed fee that is fair market value for services rendered, rather than a percentage of cost savings for their gainsharing plan. However they must ensure that those personal service contracts fall within the "safe harbor" exceptions provided by the OIG, where the payment is made in the context of a "principal-agent" relationship. Under this safe harbor, remuneration does not include any payment made by a principal to an agent as compensation for the services of the agent, as long as certain standards and conditions are met.

OTHER PARTNERSHIP POSSIBILITIES

In light of these developments, healthcare executives and physicians can benefit from examining other partnership approaches to physician pay. With the right planning and application, these plans may provide the flexibility and financial stability so highly sought after in today's market.

In developing approaches to physician pay, organization executives and physicians need to ask "What will work for us here?" In answering this question, they need to take a realistic look at the challenges associated with the plan's operation.

Most plans revolve around either the physician hospital organizations (PHO) or the management services organization (MSO). The PHO is a contracting vehicle designed to integrate hospitals with their affiliated medical staffs. Typically initiated by the hospital, the PHO's success depends largely on the strength of the physician leadership.

The MSO provides practice management services to physicians. This entity can be:

- An operating entity that owns one or more practices (a practice MSO).
- A nonoperating entity that exists to sign managed care contracts for an affiliated provider group (contracting MSO).
- Some hybrid of the two.

PHOs and MSOs both sound good on paper, but can succeed only if they do the kind of planning necessary for success. To be successful, these partnerships must engender a shared vision, develop an appropriate balance of power, agree on how to share risk and return and measure contributions to value, and spend the time necessary planning for integration. They must also provide optimal operational infrastructure, as well as develop confidence among payers for contracting purposes. Although crucial components for business success, they are rarely seen in these arrangements.

Additionally, PHOs are most likely to succeed in smaller, high-use markets with a single hospital or health system. Even then, they usually require financial restructuring at some point to resolve disputes over allocation of diminishing premium dollars. In markets with only one or two payers (the classic one-company town), payers tend to dominate the contracting climate. This situation has historically permitted little risk sharing between providers and payers. Furthermore, although physicians are critical to the survival of hospitals (by controlling what and where care is given), hospitals are not required for physician networks, and physicians are becoming increasingly wary of their involvement with PHOs. Add the gainsharing provisions previously mentioned, and it becomes clear that the strategic partnership universe must be expanded to include some new ideas.

One such new idea is the "free agent" approach. Long-term contracts have their place, but in the PHO context, they mean accepting fixed payments that then have to be redistributed among the physician partners in a PHO. Therefore, hospitals may wish to consider negotiating as "free-agent" contractors with payers, meaning they negotiate separate contracts for hospital and physician services.

Another set of ideas centers around medical settings that are independent of a large healthcare system. Indeed, the conventional wisdom regarding the utility and value of highly integrated systems is losing steam in the current market. For one thing, it is increasingly difficult to attract full risk, capitated lives from insurers on a case-rate basis. That is, payers are more and more reluctant to pay a fixed amount to providers for the total care of their members. Furthermore, the climate of greater patient choice frowns at exclusive contracts with integrated systems. As a result of these trends, some physicians are moving to work in the acute care setting, or the facility-based outpatient arena, concentrating on a particular service line, such as cardiovascular services.

Designing a compensation package to take advantage of this commercial evolution must begin with the identification or development of physicians who have a number of important traits. The physicians most suited for these new models will be genuinely interested in managing care, willing to assert strong leadership positions, capable of solving internal practice-based problems internally, and comfortable with control of protocol, utilization, and quality policies. Alliances with these physicians should offer them appropriate equity positions in the venture, aligning the entity's missions and goals with those of the physician group, and allowing physicians a strong voice in the compensation plan and the performance evaluation mechanism.

Based on the above "baseline" of an empowered, aware, commercially competent physician staff, several options exist.

- A *shared risk pool* marked by a fair and realistic per diem rate for physicians and cost-based rates for other services can give the physicians meaningful control over hospital costs and the timing of their reimbursement.
- Another such idea is the *health partnership,* which requires minimal capital. This type of entity has no physical presence, but through legal agreements (including the formation of a limited liability company) it can develop many functional

capabilities. Options include providing the clinical leadership required for service lines, performing contracting and marketing functions, and spearheading quality improvement programs such as protocol development. Parties share risks and rewards related to service line performance through incentive payments to physicians, gainsharing, or capital investments for savings arrangements.

- Yet another model is the *ambulatory services development company*, designed to own, operate, and develop new ambulatory services based on an alliance between physicians and the hospital. The physicians contribute cash, services, or technology (as permitted by law), and the hospital contributes outpatient services, facilities, and ownership responsibility.

In addition, there is the option of a *hospital-based service line management*.

- A *service line management company* created by a hospital and its physicians for management purposes is marked by capital contributions from both partners, and the provision of a fee from the hospital to manage day-to-day operations.
- This is in contrast to the *service line operating company* formed to acquire and operate both the inpatient and outpatient operations of an entire service line. Each partner retains existing ownership of facilities and equipment, strives to completely integrate management and facilities, and pursues both these dimensions to maximize its competitive advantage.
- An *integrated service line operation* is when physicians and the hospital service line merges to create an integrated service that owns, operates and develops the full service line. This venture has both parties contribute all assets, and split the rewards.

Another option might be called the PHP "pod." In this situation, the doctors organized themselves into an independent provider association (IPA) that was shaped into a "pod" structure.

In this virtual organization, specialists grouped themselves into pods by specialty and primary care doctors grouped themselves into pods of six to eight each. Each pod had its own budget and different types of incentive plans. Primary care physicians had a choice of pods based on their comfort with risk assumption, which ranged from a pure fee-for-service pod to capitated pods with varying levels of risk and commensurate potential for financial reward.

Clearly, many viable options do exist. The only question to ask is "Will this work for us here?" The answer is more likely to be yes if you can also answer in the affirmative to the five questions about incentives posed earlier in this chapter. That is, the plan should motivate the right behaviors and drive high-quality patient outcomes, physicians should understand the plan, the plan should reward nonfinancial as well as financial outcomes, and the plan should satisfy providers.

Strategic awareness, creativity, vision, and a little chutzpah can all help to deliver these requirements.

ETHICAL DESIGN PRINCIPLES

Even the best of plans require a strong ethical component, which means first and foremost that the compensation plan should prevent any conflicts of interest. Such conflicts would include any element that may impair a physician's clinical judgment and effort in ways that may benefit the provider while compromising the care received by an individual patient. This ethical imperative should be a nonnegotiable aspect of any compensation redesign effort.

Capitated compensation systems have an innate potential to cause conflicts of interest, unless the physician's pay arrangement is carefully designed. Indeed, one might say that an essential conflict of interest exists at the very "heart" of capitation, because it potentially incentivizes the witholding of necessary and appropriate care. To understand how capitated systems transmit conflict of interest, one can refer to Table 8.1. These dimensions can be used as principles to guide the development and operation of ethical capitated compensation systems.

INCENTIVES IN PHYSICIAN PAY: FIVE TRAITS TO AVOID

In designing incentives, organizations should avoid intensity, immediacy, targeting, negativity, and unfairness. The following section explains how to avoid these pitfalls.

Avoiding Intensity of Incentives

Incentives should be proportionate to the scope of services included in the agreement. They should not have too great a degree of what the medical literature calls "intensity," that is, they should not have the capability of being so large as to be out of proportion to service rendered. To avoid intensity in their incentives, healthcare organizations can provide "stop-loss" protection, a limit on the financial risk faced by physicians in caring for patients whose medical costs are unusually high. They can also control the structure, timing, and amount of any bonuses or deductions ("withholds") that are part of the risk-based plan. Caveat: Bonuses and withheld amounts that are paid out in lump sums when a specific target is attained can create conflicts of interest if the physician is close to qualifying for the extra money near the end of a contract period.

The scope of services used to calculate compensation also determines whether physicians are at any true financial risk. For example, if the costs of referral services are covered directly out of the risk pool in which the referring physician participates, physicians are truly "at risk" and, they may stand to gain or lose a lot of money, depending on how much they spend on care.

Table 8.1: Characteristics of Financial Incentives and Corresponding Design Principles for Capitated Physician-Compensation Systems

Characteristic	Design Principle

Intensity
  Scope of services
  Amount of money
  Structure of "withholds"
   and bonuses
  Stop-loss provisions
	Capitated compensation systems should not involve financial risk or gain for individual physicians that is so great as to lead reasonable persons to question whether physicians' judgments are improperly influenced.

Immediacy
  Number of physicians
  Number of patients
	Capitation should be selected as a method of compensating physicians only for large numbers of enrollees and only if there are methods available to diffuse the risk of financial loss or gain throughout a large group of physicians.

Targeting	Financial incentives should not directly reward the decreased use of specific services unless (1) there is evidence of inappropriate use of those services, (2) there are evidence-based guidelines enabling physicians to use the services more appropriately, and (3) the services are monitored for underuse.
Balance	The short-term financial incentive to use fewer services that is inherent in capitated compensation systems should be balanced by incentives that encourage physicians to incur the clinical costs necessary for excellent prevention, patient satisfaction, and clinical outcomes.
Fairness	Capitated compensation systems should make adequate allowance for clinical risk and severity in assessing and rewarding physicians' performance.

Source: Pearson, S. D., J. E. Sabin, and E. J. Emmanuel. 1998. "Ethical Guidelines for Physician Compensation Based on Capitation." *The New England Journal of Medicine* 339 (10): 689–93.

Those designing compensation plans should try to avoid financial risks or gains for individual physicians that would lead reasonable persons—for example, among patients and the general public—to question whether the physicians' judgments are improperly influenced.

Avoiding Immediacy of Incentives

Immediacy should be avoided. If intensity measures the potential size of an incentive's impact, immediacy measures the speed of that impact. The best way to blunt immediacy is to spread financial risk and gain. When the risk or gain is spread among many patients and physicians, the effect of any single medical decision on the personal income of an individual physician diminishes, reducing the potential for conflicts of interest that threaten patient trust.

Risk-based agreements covering small groups of enrollees can heighten conflicts of interest, because many of the counterbalances and safeguards that can be incorporated into payment arrangements for larger groups (e.g., stop-loss provisions) become impractical to design and implement on a smaller scale. In addition, capitation agreements involving small groups or solo practitioners may not provide enough capital to stimulate the restructuring of care.

Therefore, to build adequate safeguards into a capitation agreement, and to keep the conflict of interest to an acceptable level, the number of enrollees covered by the agreement should be larger than 250. For similar reasons, it seems reasonable to recommend that groups of physicians bearing risk should have at least 75 members.

Avoiding Targeting of Incentives

Targeting—when capitation agreements use deductions or bonuses to target specific costs for reduction—should also be avoided. Narrowly targeted incentives, such as those that focus exclusively on specific procedures such as Caesarean section, will increase the potential conflict of interest for physicians making decisions for individual patients.

Incentive-based compensation systems should not narrowly target specific services unless there is evidence of overuse of those services. Narrowly targeted incentives should be accompanied by evidence-based guidelines to help physicians determine how to use a test or treatment more appropriately, avoiding both under-use and overuse. Without such guidelines, narrowly targeted incentives can reduce the quality of care, and raise valid questions about the basis of physicians' decisions.

Avoiding Negativity of Incentives

Some incentive plans can be too negative—focusing only on reducing costs, and not on enhancing quality. The best incentive plans include specific incentives for physicians to enhance the quality of care by meeting positive goals. Such goals can counterbalance any short-term financial incentives that the physicians may have to reduce care. Many agreements reward physicians financially for ensuring patients' rapid access to care, and for achieving targets in terms of prevention and patient satisfaction. Balancing incentives can still have real financial influence and can send a clear message that physicians' compensation will not be increased solely through reduction of the use of services.

Avoiding Unfairness in Incentives

Incentives should be fair. If incentive plans shift financial risk to individual physicians without making any attempt to adjust for the clinical severity of patients' conditions and future health risks, physicians will have a built-in incentive to attract and keep only the healthiest, and therefore the least expensive, patients. This is clearly unacceptable.

Unfortunately, however, there are currently no validated, easily used methods to account for the riskiness and severity of the health of patient populations. This lack of an adequate "risk adjuster" limits the actuarial precision of capitation payments, thus penalizing physicians and groups of physicians who care for sicker patients, and rewarding those who do not.

To avoid such unfairness, organizations might consider using historical clinical data on patient groups to adjust capitation payments for risk and severity. Even subjective assessments of severity may need to be considered in setting capitation rates.

Until such risk adjusters can be developed and implemented widely, the fairness of capitated compensation systems will remain a key ethical concern. Groups of physicians that accept capitation must be vigilant in buffering individual physicians from the effects of adverse selection. It is ethically unacceptable for any system of incentives to discourage physicians from caring for the patients who are most in need.

ENCOURAGING PREVENTION

This discussion of incentives naturally leads to the subject of prevention—which is too often treated as the ancillary to healthcare, when it should be central. A major irony of capitated healthcare is the one-sided economics of preventative care—in which physicians bear the brunt of cost, with no commensurate reward. Plans value preventative care as an effective method to control costs and as a means to foster growth. They often compile what is called a "health plan employer data and information set" (HEDIS), turning it into a report card. This data includes information on how often physicians or other health professionals administer flu shots to the elderly, provide eye exams to diabetics, advise smokers to quit, prescribe beta-blockers to patients who have undergone an acute myocardial infarction (MI), and screen women for breast and cervical cancer. Plans then try to parlay good HEDIS scores into more subscribers. Therefore physicians are under increasing pressure to provide more of these services at the risk of "withholds" or even deselection from HMO networks, if their HEDIS scores audits indicate poor delivery of certain prevention services.

However, *most health plans do not reimburse for preventative services*. Furthermore, their use of administrative data may not effectively quantify the care that physicians must provide. Some studies suggest that administrative audits may underestimate physician's services by as much as 50 percent. In any event, the HEDIS measure certainly fails to account for the time-consuming and difficult nature of delivering preventative services. Consequently much of the effort to promote wellness comes at the physician's expense.

The combination of prevention goals and lack of preventive care reimbursement is creating an impossible situation for physicians. They are being asked to spend less time with each patient and to fit more prevention practice time into each visit for the same basic reimbursements dollar, with the spectre of stiff penalties if this is not done appropriately. This is a huge disincentive that must be counterbalanced in any compensation plan.

A financial incentive should be engineered into any plan to reward providers for delivering prevention measures at a high rate. For this to have any relevance, providers should be given sufficient tools to enable tracking of patients and to ensure regular follow-up for preventative testing, education, and counseling.

Additionally, more pressure must be placed on health plans and Medicare to promote preventative practices. Plans and Medicare should reimburse providers fairly for services provided under federal guidelines. Any physician that provides healthcare services covered under current procedural terminology (CPT) codes accepted by the Centers for Medicare & Medicaid Services (the agency that administers Medicare and Medicaid), should reward physicians for counseling almost as much as it should for a midlevel office visit. This incentive must be in place throughout the health-care industry.

In the interim, it may make sense for practices to have patients pay for care that is not reimbursed. This may seem distasteful at first blush to many providers. However, evidence shows that patients who pay out of pocket for prevention may be more likely to comply with a weight loss or smoking cessation program. If patients spend their own money on such a program, rather than a health plan's money, they may take actually take the preventative steps their physician recommends. Since this is the real goal of prevention, it may be a strategy worth thinking about.

IMPLEMENTING AND SUPPORTING THE COMPENSATION PLAN

Each payment method must be customized to the utilization patterns, specialty, and practice behaviors of individual physicians. Also, the method must be supported by accurate and timely information and financial systems. Having physicians who are truly integrated and dependent on one another is also critical to success.

CONCLUSION

In this chapter, we have seen a number of models that can ensure appropriate pay for physicians. The most important component of a physician compensation plan is to form a good match between the quality of care and the generosity of reward. Physicians should have incentives to avoid overuse of unnecessary services, and to encourage use of necessary services. This means no more readmissions to an acute care bed because of an inaccessible physician, no more trips to the emergency room for minor illnesses, and no more overuse of unnecessary and costly procedures. All these must become anathema for a compensation plan to have any chance of survival.

Additionally, physicians and their organizations must design supporting information systems to be sophisticated enough to generate real-time reports to identify and rectify inappropriate utilization patterns before so much time has passed that the point is moot and the capitated budget exhausted. Systems must be capable of tracking patients by physician, by diagnosis, and by payer. In this way, through risk assessment and intervention, physicians can anticipate and prevent potential health problems and complications within their practices. They can also ensure equitable risk sharing.

Most importantly, physicians must understand their compensation plan in its entirety. After all, physicians are the ultimate drivers of improved quality of care, and the ultimate recipients of any financial rewards that will be generated by this improvement. Organizations and their advisors should include key medical leadership early in the process, not only bringing compensation ideas to physicians, but also on assisting, advising, and guiding them to make behavioral changes required to meet all practice goals. Physicians are by nature independent, intelligent, and strong-willed, and comprehensive compensation plans require collaboration, teamwork, and flexibility. Medical leaders must therefore assume the role of team leaders and facilitators in making the link between care cost and quality.

Finally, the "right" compensation plan must be defined and shaped by physicians because they will live and work under it, with both financial and professional effects. All involved parties should seek to craft a compensation plan that offers appropriate incentives, discourages conflicts of interest, and rewards preventative care. Such a plan offers a rational, acceptable, and effective method to manage both care and costs and put control back in the hands of physicians and patients. Indeed, such a plan will motivate physicians to take the lead in developing new systems and protocols required for more effective care management.

NOTE

1. Dr. Regina Herzlinger has written extensively on the subject of market-driven healthcare, noting its benefits and drawbacks. For a recent article outlining her research and similar findings, see Paul Goodyear, "Managing a Good Cause," *CMA Management Magazine,* December/January 2001. Mr. Goodyear is the assistant financial secretary of the Salvation Army.

REFERENCES

Gaynor M, and P. Gertler. 1995. "Moral Hazard and Risk Spreading in Partnerships." *RAND Journal of Economics* 26 (4): 591–613.

Office of the Inspector General (OIG). 1999. "Special Advisory Bulletin." U.S. Health and Human Services. Washington, DC: OIG. July 8.

Pearson, S. D., J. E. Sabin, and E. J. Emmanuel. 1998. "Ethical Guidelines for Physician Compensation Based on Capitation." *The New England Journal of Medicine* 339 (10): 689–93.

U.S. General Accounting Office (GAO). 1986. "Medical Physician Incentive Payments by Hospitals Could Lead to Abuse." Washington, DC: GAO. July 1.

CHAPTER 9

Establishing Positive Media Relations: A Guide for Hospital CEOs and Directors

Bruce M. Meyer and Eileen Rochford

TODAY'S HEALTHCARE CEOS can face a barrage of criticism over salary. Recent headlines tell the story:

"County Bailout of Hospital Raises Questions Over CEO's Salary"

The Washington Post, June 7, 2001

"Hospital Execs Got Raises As Cuts Came; . . . Hospitals, But Not Their Execs, Struggled"

Post-Standard, May 5, 2001

"Two Hospitals Struggle, But Not Top Execs"

Associated Press Newswires, May 8, 2001

". . . Health Care Professionals Dissent over Rising Salaries"

Standard-Examiner, July 4, 2001

What can a responsible CEO and board of directors do to ensure that stories like this do not put their hospitals in an unfavorable light?

SCENARIO 1

It is 5:15, and the phone of the local hospital has been ringing off the hook all day long. There it goes again! The CEO picks it up.

The person on the line identifies herself as a reporter with the local ABC television affiliate. "My research department just gave me a copy of your hospital's 990 form," the reporter explains. "Based on the figures on this form, your earnings for the last year were $470,000. In light of your hospital's recent layoffs, how can you justify your salary?"

The CEO responds indignantly: "This hospital was hemorrhaging cash before I came here, and I staunched the flow. The hospital is lucky there weren't more layoffs—there would have been if I hadn't come along! And as for my pay, I earned every penny of it—and at the going market rate, based on surveys, I am paid at the 60th percentile of salaries for CEOs of hospitals of this size and area of the country."

The reporter quotes sound bites from the CEO on the 6:00 news that evening. "Hemorrhaging cash . . . , lucky there weren't more layoffs . . . earned every penny." The CEO's words are taken out of context—juxtaposed with other material in the most unflattering way. Media coverage spreads to all of the local stations and continues for days. Soon there is a massive local outcry and calls for the CEO's resignation. The hospital goes on the defensive and stays there, with long-lasting repercussions.

SCENARIO 2

The CEO's phone rings at 5:15 p.m. This time, the call is routed to the hospital's public relations (PR) department. The representative from the department exchanges pleasantries with the reporter and reminds her that the chairman of the compensation committee is the only person who can comment on reported salaries. The PR representative asks the reporter what her deadline is, and learns that it is close of business the following day. Taking care to meet the reporter's deadline, the PR person immediately calls the chairman of the compensation committee to arrange an interview the following day at noon. Prior to the interview, the PR team meets with the chairman to coach her on proper responses, which were developed well in advance of this particular inquiry. The team also discusses possible and probable follow-up questions, and practices interview role-playing with the chairman to make sure she is as prepared as possible.

When the story airs that evening, the reporter shows footage of the hospital and what its new management has accomplished over the past year. Her report explains that hospitals compete heavily for qualified leaders, and provides local and national market compensation data to illustrate the point. The story includes background from prior meetings the hospital has held with the media following board meetings. The report does include sound bites complaining about the CEO's "rich" salary, but, all in all, it is a well-rounded story. The community reaction is mild—even positive —and the story receives no further coverage.

A CHOICE

Imagine yourself in the shoes of either of these CEO s. Which one would you rather be?

The likelihood that you will be faced with a similar situation in the near future has increased dramatically in the last three years. Stories that feature the publishing of local hospital CEO salaries are now almost commonplace—and the after-effects of this type of news coverage can be devastating. How you prepare for and handle working with the media can mean the difference between the first scenario and the second. Now more than ever, your reputation can hinge upon your relationship with your local newspapers, television, and radio stations.

HOSPITAL CEOS IN THE NEWS

The following examples—all covered by the media in 2001—illustrate examples of coverage of hospital CEO compensation packages, both positive and negative. These stories are useful to keep in mind when outlining a public relations strategy for handling this type of media coverage or inquiry, and especially useful if a hospital has experienced any types of performance problems in recent years. Reporters will be especially attuned to these issues, and will tie them back to any questions regarding CEO compensation increases.

Consider the case of a highly regarded CEO of a mid-sized hospital in a northeastern city. This CEO was awarded a 31 percent increase in salary and benefits by the hospital's board in April 2001. The resulting coverage of this news cited the CEO's performance, and compared his compensation package favorably with top executives at other midsized hospitals.

The local newspaper included quotes from the chairman of the board, who said of the CEO, "We don't want to lose this man; he is very good." The article also detailed the CEO's contributions to the hospital, describing the major role he played not only in the physical expansions at the hospital, but also in its expanding services throughout the community. The story received exactly one day of news coverage, and the CEO's generous raise quickly became a non-issue.

A similar media success story unfolded in February 2001 for another hospital CEO in a southeastern city. This CEO was hired for a hefty sum, and the local newspaper covered the news of the hiring, reporting the amount of the CEO's incoming salary. The CEO's contract, which a board member called "standard," called for him to make $280,000 per year. In a well-planned interview with the local newspaper, the vice chairman of the board explained that for each year of his contract, the CEO will earn between 15 and 30 percent of his base salary if he meets or exceeds short-term performance goals. The vice chairman of the board was also quoted in the story: "The way the system is designed, the better the hospital does, the better this person does." This article was the first and last on the subject; the CEO's raise resulted in only one day of coverage.

Also instructive is the case of a pair of Southwestern hospitals— including one that U.S. News & World Report recently rated among the top 50 specialized hospitals in the U.S. Both hospitals have recently undergone financial hardship. Neither hospital implemented an effective PR plan to communicate CEO salary increases to the public, and both hospitals paid dearly for it in the form of negative media coverage.

One hospital's story came out in February 2001, sparking a barrage of negatively slanted articles that ran in the local city newspapers until July 2001. It all began on February 16, when the main local newspaper reported that the board of directors at one of the hospitals was considering giving its CEO a 4 percent raise in salary. Members of the local city council began protesting the decision in light of the hospital's recent financial difficulties—even though the local city council had no authority over hospital salaries.

Two days after the first story broke, the same newspaper came out with a second article that quoted hospital employees who resented the proposed pay raise for the CEO. They protested that rank-and-file salaries at the institution had been frozen for years. Because of the negative media coverage, the vote on the CEO's salary was indefinitely postponed.

But PR disasters did not stop there. In April, the other hospital quietly granted its CEO a 13 percent annual salary increase during a late-night board meeting, without announcing the increase to the public. The next month, the story broke in the local paper. Reaction was both swift and negative. Several council members said the raise was both poorly timed and unnecessary, considering the hospital had failed to make a profit for two years and had recently announced plans to begin charging patients for parking.

After months of argument between the hospital board and the city council, the council voted to take back powers of salary decision making from the hospital board. This set off a firestorm of legal debate and activity, all of which was reported extensively in the local media. In July, an article quoted a councilman who said that all this could have been avoided "had more attention been paid to public relations." Furthermore, a hospital board member told the newspaper that it could take "years" for the board to recover from the damage that the controversy did to its image.

Considering the inopportune timing of these raises, the hospitals should have put more PR effort into announcing them. Better communication between the hospitals, local governing bodies, and employees may not have solved the hospitals' compensation problems, but it could have lessened them considerably.

LESSONS LEARNED—ADVICE FROM HOSPITAL CEOS

Hospital CEOs who have weathered compensation crises can testify to the importance of good constituency relations. That is the firm conviction of Howard Chase, president and CEO for Methodist Hospital of Dallas. After 35 years in the industry, he firmly believes that how news reporters treat his hospital during crisis periods is due in large part to the steps he has taken to serve their needs.

"We make a great effort to hold quarterly meetings with local reporters," says Chase. "While we go into those meetings with points we wanted to get across, we intentionally leave them open for plenty of Q&A so that reporters will feel they have a chance to steer the conversations as well. It doesn't work to just push out information. In order to have a good working relationship with reporters, you have to be willing to respond to their needs and interests."

Chase recalls what happened when Methodist Hospital reported his salary.

"I didn't get any press calls regarding my salary. Our PR department handled all the calls, using the statement and other preparations that we had made in anticipation of questions like that. They cited third-party stats on salary ranges in the industry and allowed the chairman of our board to answer questions. It was maybe a two-day story and was relatively harmless."

Chase hastens to add that preparing statements is not the same thing as bending the truth. "Being open and honest with reporters—always—is paramount," he declares. "I think we've done a good job of not trying to put a snow job on any story, good or bad, over the years. That serves us well, especially in times of real crisis. The media knows that we are telling the truth no matter what the issue, since we always try to give accurate and timely information, no matter what the circumstances."

Of course, communication cannot carry the entire burden, Chase notes. It is important to "make the right choices for your community" in the first place. Sometimes, however, there will be bad news. Hospitals should "make a point to communicate regularly with local media about both the good and the bad," he says. "If you do that, you'll be treated much more fairly when the darts start flying."

Chase and his staff go through training to prepare for media interviews approximately every two years, although he feels that might not be often enough in today's media environment. This year, the hospital accelerated the process when it hired a new director of public relations.

Another CEO, Eugene Leblond, who recently took on a position with Pocono Health Systems in Pennsylvania, has strong opinions on how to handle media questions about executive salaries.

"It creates a lot of difficulty when a CEO's salary and benefits are put out there and it is considerably higher than the rest of the workforce," says Leblond. "I have seen a lot of newspaper headlines from my colleagues who have handled it well and not so well recently. I think it's an issue of being aware and prepared."

While Leblond has not personally experienced negative press coverage as a result of having his salary reported, he says his PR staff is well prepared in the event that it should come up.

"When I got here, I was so impressed that the PR team had created a crisis communications manual," says Leblond. "It includes a checklist of various scenarios that might happen, with the proper procedures to follow. If something happens here and we need to get the press the right information, we know what to do." The manual, which is updated at least once per year, maps out responses to typical scenarios including breach of confidentiality, celebrity patients, executive turnover, mass casualty, medical malpractice, and communicable diseases. Leblond praises the manual's utility: "This is all ready right now so that if we have a disaster, we can respond quickly. It has worked very well for us."

Leblond agrees that developing a relationship with local press can be the key to achieving a balanced story. "Reporters need to understand that you are being open and honest with them and I think the best way to do that is to develop a rapport on the front end if you can," he says.

Leblond remembers that when he came on board, the hospital had had a difficult relationship with the press for about 10 years. He told the staff that he planned to be open and honest with the press from the start, laying all cards on the table—including information about unpopular (and possibly bad) board decisions. The reaction from the staff was overwhelmingly negative. They believed that the media would scrutinize every bit of information shared, in search of the most negative aspects to report. Following the first board meeting under his watch, Leblond proceeded as planned by sharing all information with the local media. Admittedly, this first experience was difficult—resulting in about 30 questions that directors themselves could not answer. Fortunately, however, the staff was able to provide the additional information needed. Subsequent coverage of board meetings was largely positive, he says.

"I think we in healthcare sometimes tend to try to hide information or try to get 100 percent of the information before responding to reporters. In times of crisis that will not work," insists Leblond. "The better route is evaluating what information you do have and determining what makes sense to share as the situation transpires. Above all, make sure what you are sharing is accurate."

See Figure 9.1 for helpful tips from both Chase and Leblond on how to discuss compensation information with the media.

Figure 9.1: Communicating Compensation Information: Ten Tips from CEOs

1. Actively tell your story on an ongoing basis.
2. Be prepared for all possible scenarios; don't get caught unprepared.
3. Develop a relationship with your local media through meetings and open houses.
4. Channel all media calls through the PR department.
5. Let the board chairman or chairman of the compensation committee act as spokesperson, not the CEO.
6. Be sensitive to the needs of media; meet deadlines.
7. Be timely, not waiting for 100 percent of the information before communicating.
8. Be forthright, giving information fully.
9. Be honest, giving information accurately.
10. Don't hide the bad news—and make sure the good news is known.

THE MEDIA LANDSCAPE

The mass media—newspapers, radio, television, and even the Internet—provide valuable opportunities to deliver the messages of a healthcare institution to the local community and beyond. There are basically three ways to access these media: advertisements, articles, and interviews.

Advertisements—sound bites, clips, or publication space purchased by a healthcare institution—offer control over content, but they often carry a significant cost. Furthermore, although they can be influential, they are considered a less desirable way to communicate than through "editorial" offerings.

Articles—ranging from lengthy articles in medical journals to short "op-eds" in newspapers—also offer some degree of control, and their cost is variable. If a hospital executive has already been writing on a topic, and finds a friendly publication, placement and publication requires little time or expense. On the other hand, if an institution aspires to place an article or op-ed in a sought-after publication with very high circulation and a low acceptance rate, working toward article publication can be a costly and occasionally fruitless (not every letter to the editor or op-ed gets published.)

In comparison to advertisements and articles, submission to interviews can seem like a high-impact, low-cost route. Interviews, however, do have their pitfalls. First, it is not always possible to get a journalist interested in conducting an interview. Second, when the journalist does consent to interview, the desire to conduct the interview may be focused around some problem area, rather than a successful one. These hurdles can be overcome, however, with the proper interview guidance.

INTERVIEW GUIDANCE

It is helpful to understand the perspectives of journalists before working with them. A journalist's business is to inform, to analyze, and to comment. Consequently, journalists are not interested in merely reproducing generally known facts or in presenting a neutral portrait of your company or industrial sector. Instead, they are interested in telling an interesting story and illustrating it with a variety of different—even clashing—viewpoints. Journalists depend on those who supply them with information. Hospital leaders can fill that information need and in doing so, build a beneficial relationship.

If you are a hospital senior manager or director, you may find yourself, as the designated spokesperson of your institution, speaking about compensation. In such a case, in addition to the "Ten Tips" from CEOs, it is important to know some of the "dos and don'ts" PR professionals can offer from decades of hard experience (see Figure 9.2).

Figure 9.2: Dos and Don'ts

Don't try to handle everything yourself.
Do work with your PR department to determine who from the organization should be speaking about what issues, and then let your staff know these names and their contact information so they can forward calls as appropriate.

Don't agree to an interview if you feel uncomfortable about it.
Do postpone the interview until you feel a level of comfort.

Don't let yourself be pressured by deadlines.
Do try to respect deadlines, but always ask if they can be moved; and remember, a bad interview is worse than no interview at all.

Don't let reporters control the interview.
Do be obliging and friendly, but set interview boundaries with confidence.

Don't assume that you have the upper hand with respect to all undisclosed inside information.
Do remember that there is always the potential for an information "leak."

Don't improvise.
Do think about what messages you want to get across in your interview, and incorporate these messages into your answers right from the start.

Don't "save the best for last."
Do be sure to make your most important points upfront in the conversation.
(If you wait, you may not get time to deliver them if the conversation is curtailed.)

Don't be vague.
Do make clear statements.

Don't speculate.
Do stick to the facts you know for certain. A phrase such as "I'm not sure but I can try to find out for you" is always better than dancing around the subject.

Don't speak only for yourself personally.
Do familiarize yourself with the official viewpoint of your institution and represent that first and foremost. If you have a personal view, make sure to express it as just that.

Don't let yourself be provoked into responding emotionally.
Do stick to the facts you prepared.

Don't ramble.
Do stick to the topic the journalist is interested in; journalists too, have very little time.

Don't agree to an interview on the spot when reporters catch you off guard with a surprise phone call.
Do ask to call them back, which will allow you time to talk with your PR person and ensure you time to relax and focus on the interview.

Don't get sandbagged.
Do make sure your PR department or agency does some digging on the reporter and the interview topic before you go into your interview.

CONCLUSION

By following the dos and don'ts offered by public relations professional, as well as the other advice provided in this chapter, healthcare leaders can turn interactions with the press into opportunities—for both themselves and their organizations.

REFERENCES

Chase, H. 2001. Interview with author, July 19.

Leblond, E. 2001 Interview with author, July 20.

Epilogue

IN THE PAST nine chapters, the contributors to this book have presented some of the main features of healthcare compensation—from setting policy elements in the boardroom, to building positive media relations in the "pressroom." Chapters have also covered a variety of technical subjects, such as the latest IRS rulings for disclosing pay in not-for-profits, and intricacies of designing a physician pay plan or analyzing an employment contract.

In developing this book, the contributors had a collective goal: to make the subject of executive compensation less mysterious. Trustees and executives should have the ability to understand and address this subject with the information necessary to make an informed decision.

Whatever information you needed, we trust that this book has delivered it. If you have further questions, contact me (tpflannery@hotmail.com) and I will try to help. Conversely, if you would like to share your expertise in future editions of this book, let me know. I will add you to my roster of distinguished contributors.

Joining now with my contributors, I hereby thank you for your attention. I wish you all success in setting and maintaining sound compensation programs in your healthcare organization now and in the future.

About the Authors

CHAPTER 1

Thomas P. Flannery, PH.D., is a partner with the Andersen Human Capital practice. Based in Boston, he serves as competency leader of Andersen's People Strategy and Human Resource Management Group in the United States. He is the author of *People, Performance, and Pay* (Simon & Schuster's Free Press 1996). He has also published numerous articles about compensation in healthcare and other fields. He holds a B.A. in education from Arizona State University, an M.A. in public administration from the University of New Mexico, and a PH.D. in administration and social policy from Northwestern University.

CHAPTER 2

Thomas P. Flannery, PH.D.

Deborah (Debbie) L. Rose is a manager in the Human Capital Practice of Andersen. She assists organizations in a variety of areas, from compensation plan design to human resource process redesign. Her experience includes a wide range of industries and spans from small, privately held companies to large corporations. She earned a B.B.A from the University of Massachusetts in human resource management and has P.H.R. designation from the Society of Human Resource Management. She is currently pursuing her M.B.A. at Boston College. She is also pursuing her certified compensation professional (CCP) designation through the American Compensation Association. In addition, Debbie is a member of the Society for Human Resource Management (SHRM) and the Northeast Human Resource Association (NEHRA).

CHAPTER 3

James A. Landry, PH.D., a partner with the Andersen Human Capital practice, is based in Houston, Texas. He has over two decades of consulting experience, including work with major corporations in compensation and change management. He serves on the faculty of the University of Houston Graduate School of Business. Dr. Landry attended Cornell University and Wagner College (B.A.) for his undergraduate studies. He received his M.A. from New York University and a PH.D. in counseling psychology from the University of Texas School of Public Health. He received his B.A. degree from Columbia College in New York City and his M.D. degree from Boston University School of Medicine.

Ralph D. Feigin, M.D., is the J.S. Abercrombie professor of pediatrics and chairman of the department of pediatrics at the Baylor College of Medicine and physician-in-chief of the Texas Children's Hospital. In addition, he is physician-in-chief, pediatric service, Ben Taub General Hospital (Harris County District), and chief of the pediatric service, The Methodist Hospital, Houston, Texas.

CHAPTER 4

Diane Cornwell is a tax partner in the Louisville office of Andersen and serves as the firm's national director of the Tax-Exempt and Higher Education Tax Practices and a member of the firm's National Healthcare Team. Her experience includes physician relationships, reorganizations, compensation, intermediate sanctions, tax-exempt status, inurement of benefit, joint venture participation, and acquisition structuring. Diane graduated with "highest distinction" from Indiana University's Kelley School of Business with a B.S. She is a licensed certified public accountant.

Christine Jha, based in Louisville, is a tax manager specializing in tax-exempt organizations. She advises her clients on a variety of matters including compensation, tax compliance, tax-exempt status, unrelated business income, and IRS exam planning. Christine holds a B.A. from Bellarmine University and is a certified public accountant.

CHAPTER 5

Jeffrey D. Frank is a senior manager in the Andersen Human Capital practice in Indianapolis, where he specializes in retirement income plans and executive compensation. He brings over a decade of experience to Andersen's national team, specializing in compensation matters for healthcare and other tax-exempt organizations. Mr. Frank holds a B.S. in business from Indiana University and an M.S. in taxation from Drexel University. He coauthored *Arthur Andersen Guide to Navigating Intermediate Sanctions* (Jossey-Bass, 2000).

Daniel B. Kennedy is a manager in the human capital practice in Atlanta, where he specializes in compensation consulting. He has over a decade of experience in human resources and compensation matters. He holds a B.A. degree in economics and an M.B.A. from Duke University. His areas of focus in healthcare consulting include competitive pay surveys, employment agreements, reasonable compensation analyses, deferred compensation programs, and incentive plan design.

David D. Scaife is a manager in Andersen's Life Insurance Products Consulting Group in Milwaukee. Mr. Scaife is a certified public account, and has a B.S. in finance from the University of Wisconsin–Eau Claire and an M.S. in taxation from the University of Wisconsin–Milwaukee. He has extensive experience with health-care clients and specializes in transactions involving life insurance, such as the purchase of new or review of existing life insurance policies including split-dollar insurance.

CHAPTER 6

Douglas M. Mancino is a partner in McDermott, Will & Emery's Los Angeles office. He has represented all types of nonprofit organizations for more than 25 years on tax, business, and financial matters. He represents organizations and individuals in connection with the formation of nonprofit organizations such as public charities, private foundations and trade associations, corporate transactions such as mergers and acquisitions, joint ventures, shared services, conversions from nonprofit to for-profit status, and restructuring of corporate organizations. He has had extensive experience in audit, appeals, and tax controversy matters, and has served as lead tax counsel in eight audits conducted by the IRS as part of its Coordinated Examination Program for tax-exempt organizations, and has litigated several tax cases in the U.S. Tax Court and in the U. S. Court of Appeals. A widely published author of both articles and books, he is active in professional associations and serves on editorial advisory boards of three prestigious journals. Mr. Mancino received his B.A., cum laude, from Kent State University in 1971, and his J.D. degree, summa cum laude, from The Ohio State University College of Law in 1974.

CHAPTER 7

Jack Schlosser, FACHE, is a partner with Spencer Stuart in Los Angeles, where he is a member of the firm's Life Sciences practice focusing on CEO and other senior-level searches. His specialties include health systems and physician practice management, among other special fields. Mr. Schlosser is a Fellow (and former Regent) of the American College of Healthcare Executives and a past-president of the UCLA Health Services Management Alumni Association. He is a graduate of the University of California at Los Angeles, where he received an M.A. in public health in health services management, and of the United States International University, where he received a B.A. degree.

CHAPTER 8

Charles A. Peck, M.D., FACP, is a partner with Andersen based in Atlanta. He is an internist with 23 years of healthcare experience as a clinician, an administrator, and a medical director for a national managed care company. He consults with clients in the areas of integrated delivery systems, hospital operations, e-commerce, Medicare risk contracting, clinical care coordination and development, physician leadership, value creation, biotechnology, and change management. He received his B.A. from Emory University in Atlanta and his M.D. from New York University. He is also a graduate of the Case Western Reserve University's Weatherhead School of Management Professional Fellows program and the Wharton School of Management Physician Executive Training program. Dr. Peck, who is board certified in internal medicine and rheumatology, completed his residency and fellowship in internal medicine and rheumatology at University Hospitals of Cleveland.

CHAPTER 9

Bruce M. Meyer is the global director of marketing for Andersen's Human Capital practice. He joined the firm in 1996 and works out of the Atlanta office. Mr. Meyer has 20 years of experience in the marketing and management of professional service organizations and was the managing editor of the *Andersen Human Capital Book* 1996–2001 series. Mr. Meyer is also a member of the American Marketing Association, Direct Marketing Association, Society for Human Resources (SHRM), World@Work, and board member of the Atlanta Dogwood Festival. Mr. Meyer holds a Bachelor of Business Administration and a M.M.A. from the University of Georgia.

Eileen Rochford is a vice president of Ketchum, a leading public relations firm. Based in Chicago, she has counseled a variety of major companies throughout the United States. Her overall communications experience spans several disciplines, including issues management, strategic planning, public affairs, crisis communications, and marketing communications. Eileen graduated from Marquette University with Bachelor degrees in journalism and political science.

Index

Chairman (of the board): CEO as, 5, 6; compensation committee role, 4–5; function, 4; position description, 6–8; role, 6

Change management, 64–65, 67–68

Change-of-control provisions, 30, 173–174

Charter, 3, 15–16, 20

Chief executive officer (CEO): board of directors and, 2; cash compensation comparison, 49, 52, 53, 55, 57; as chairman of board, 5, 6; compensation committee, 5; media relations, 285–293; performance evaluation, 4; position description, 8–10; role, 6

Chief financial officer (CFO), 50, 52, 54, 56–57

Chief operating officer (COO), 49, 52

Choice of law provision, 179

Churning, 267

CII. See Council for Institutional Investors

Club survey, 33–34

Collaboration, 73

Collateral assignment split-dollar arrangement, 152–153, 155–156

Commitment, 73

Common cost methodology, 29

Communication, 73, 75, 89

Company representative, 8, 10

Comparable data, 122–123

Compensation: aspects, 1–2; definition, 47; elements, 33; market data, 32–38; media coverage, 285–293; negotiation, 248–250; physician. See Physician compensation; practical considerations, 31–32; reasonable determination, 108, 109–119; strategic considerations, 30–31, 42–43; survey information, 32; threshold, 32; valuation, 29–30

Compensation committee: activities, 19–20; chairman, 13–14; charter, 15–16, 20; composition, 14, 16–20; concerns, 5–6; disclosure duties, 20–22; independence, 4–6, 16–19; meetings, 7; membership, 5, 19–20; responsibilities, 20; role, 10–13

Competency: assessment form, 84, 85–86; core, 71; definition, 68; examples, 77; key characteristics, 70–71; leadership, 68, 70–75; performance indicator, 79–80

Competitive passion, 73

Competitive position, 9

Competitive practice, 41

Confidentiality, 182, 257

Conflict of interest: capitated compensation, 274–279; due care, 3–4; policy, 121, 128–134; procedures, 130; recruitment issues, 257–258; violations, 131

Contact compensation, 267

Contracting MSO, 271

Contribution allocation, 172

Controlled entities, 103

COO. See Chief operating officer

Corporate Library, 12

Council for Institutional Investors (CII), 18–19

Counseling, 280–281

Covenant not to compete, 180–181

Covey, Stephen, 72

Culture, 8–9, 60, 67, 73

Data cuts, 33

Deductibility limits, 5, 16, 17–18

Deferred compensation: advantage, 142; annual limits, 145–146; cash-based, 147–148; design considerations, 140–143; economics, 139–140; employment contract provisions, 171–172; industry trends, 46; ineligible Section 457 plans, 160–162; insurance-based arrangements, 148–160; mutual fund option plans, 162–165; non-deferral comparison, 141; Section 162 bonus plan, 149–151; split-dollar arrangements, 151–160; strategies, 137–138, 143–145

Defined benefit plan, 144

Defined contribution plan, 144

Delegation, 75

Dental insurance, 45

Disability insurance, 45

Disclosure: compensation committee, 20–22; duty, 129–130; excessive